American Sizism Sucks

by

katy glenn willis

American Sizism Sucks

Authored by Katy Glenn Willis

Copyright © 2012

ALL RIGHTS RESERVED

ISBN-10: 1479370711
ISBN-13: 9781479370719

**

Cover art by Katy Glenn Willis

Cover design by Rachel Lackey

Thank you to all who gave permission to print your songs and poems in this book.

"It is what it is,
it's
all
in
the handling."

-John Trudell

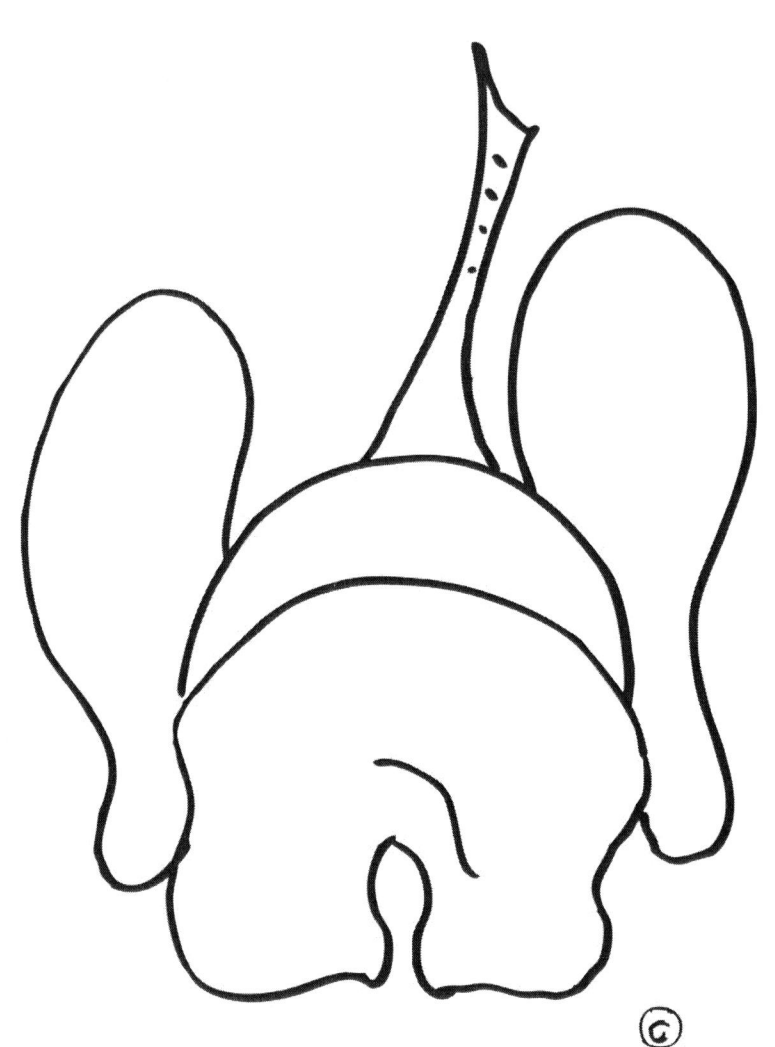

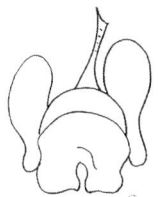

HELLO

Once upon a troubled time, in a small tennessee town where a lot of people reside who are connected to the literary and academic world, a group of us women formed a monthly gathering wherein the purpose was always evolving, but consistently included beginning with open communication about our current experiences. And so it began, one eve, with a newer member sharing the disturbing event in her day.

While enjoying the natural quiet of her rural surroundings, she was seriously shocked by turning to see a stranger on the property! It was not so much that her private time had been interrupted, she conveyed, but that the woman who approached was exceptionally large and dressed in a vibrant red outfit. With total disgust she expressed, "How did a person her size feel the right to wear a color which accentuated her presence when her size alone was enough to demand negative attention?"

OMG - no one shifted in their seat, no one seemed surprised, no one spoke out!

Having just gained thirty unwanted pounds, having spent my life inundated by size prejudices, and naturally wearing pants highlighted with red which just happens to be my favorite color, I sank into my chair, flushed (oh crap red faced) with embarrassment. I remained in this oppressed pose the duration of that agonizing evening, then without even a goodbye, slipped out, hurrying home to safety and a long sleepless night. In a flood of terrible memories, the emotional pains and anxieties overwhelmed me.

At the break of dawn, fueled by a sausage biscuit and some rising indignant inspiration, I began to write.

There are many people in this country who needlessly suffer degradation and discrimination which affects them not only socially, but also financially, plus, with tremendous force, psychologically. The words I write are to honor you who are personally stricken by sizism. Actually, any ism, since they all have the same result. Plus, hopefully to inform you who are still unaware and ignor-ant of your prejudices that the harm done is way beyond your awareness. The problem of size discrimination which has caused humans such self hatred that they shut themselves away and even commit suicide, I do declare, is no longer acceptable and shall end. No matter how righteous a belief system might seem, as many believe obesity to be acute laziness, stupidity and sloven, to judge a person to be too gross to walk the same earth as you - welp - that is downright sick. And that judgment, like any other, sucks you right in and keeps you in a place which is sucky.

YEPPERS: American Sizism Sucks! It makes an ass of all who participate.

Lots of folks in the usa have come to at least consider that racism, classism, ageism, sexism, and any other ism I forgot, are detrimental. If you really look at 'em, they are fear based. Yet we are mostly unconsciously immersed still in the socio-economic, and political, body size discrimination. It even carries into car, house, bank account, tv screen, you name it - manifestations of an opposite projection, but for now we stick with the bod as a whole since we all know the opposite attitude toward certain parts. Funny that the outer material possession size preference is directly opposite of the more personal physique. For clarification sake, it is those who are deemed FAT who are most harshly judged, tho there are some who also lay disgust upon the too skinny. Alas, in all forms of prejudice, aint one side always lookin ta find a reason ta judge, even hate, the other? And like most beliefs these days, this problem is so extreme it is politically correct, socially acceptable, and economically feasible. Talk about an unholy trinity!

We are all, no matter our background or appearance, of one simple being: we love joy; we hate pain. Tis that simple. There's plenty of pain around. Shall we continue in a mind set which undermines so many americans? The cost in loving, attention, money, and happiness is way high.
The younger ones are certainly rebelling, enlarging and accepting fat friends in even revealing attire, butt it aint over by a long shot. Models, movies, medias: sales, sales, sales. They still all accentuate the sizism systems.

Sizism sucks you right in, chews you up, and spits you out in a BIG FAT wad.

Welcome to my WORD....

and my WORLD...........

Bear with me cuz it is a dynamic experience which does all come together in an ah hah for all........

the answer

-by dafire burns

once again

i find my self……………..face down

on

the

stone
       cold
                floor

of desire.

what's that you say?

ahh yes

JUMP……. in The Fire

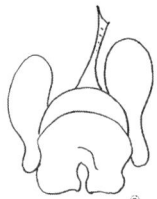

IN THE BEGINNING THERE WUZ SUGAR

It was 1950 when I was born in to this world on a beautiful fall afternoon in a small southern Appalachian town. Unlike the mountain life of my father's youth, my family purchased our meat from the grocer, bathed indoors daily, spent summers at the country club swimming pool and attended school grades K-12. In other words, I was raised an upper middle class baby boomer in a family where both parents remembered the depression, served in THE war, and enjoyed the affluence that post war times offered Caucasian Americans - even tho my Pa was dark skinned, black haired, and quite representative of the Monacan and Melungeon blood which also courses strong in my veins. We were steeped in the American Dream: parental evening cocktails followed by large home cooked family dinners attended by both parents, 2 children + one dog. It was assumed that us kids would graduate college and succeed in a career. We had safe neighborhoods, lotsa new clothes and plenty of whatever we wanted. On the exterior our life was perfect.

Travel back with me to the spring of 1953. Picture a seasonably warm, crisp, absolutely alive spring morning: leaves budding, dogwoods blooming, daffodils lining the driveways of sweet little middle class starter homes along quiet new suburban streets. I am now two and a half years along and this is my very first memory. Dressed in those terribly uncomfortable scratchy lace petticoats called crinolines, YUK!; topped by a white cotton and lace dress with pink ribbon along the waistline, and white lace lined socks inside my little patent leather covered feet; I was Easter Sunday Church ready. Consequently, the bells always adorning at least one article of my clothing were left on the dresser, leaving me un-track-able and primed for espionage style action.

Aware that both my parents and my older brother were entrenched in dressing for The Christian fashion holiday of the year, I snuck out the back door and over to the rear screen enclosed porch at our neighbor's, an elderly couple expecting little egg hunting grandchildren after church. The exciting awareness of my first pre-meditated and consciously illicit act in life was memorably plowing a lifelong neural-pathway into my little gray matter. As the adrenaline pumped my bitty bod, nerve transmissions engorged gullies in my brain; deep as in the surrounding suburban sprawl of clear-cut land when it comes a downpour. Like the mud water flow on laid bare land, I was surely on my way to seeking out many similarly unforgettable experiences.

Carrying my own Easter basket, strategically half emptied by my early morning snacking, actually gorging, I slowly crept onto the neighbor's porch. Having already cased the joint, I knew several baskets awaited the arrival of their grandkids. Full to the brim and overflowing with fake neon green plastic grass, my sought caches glistened of foil covered chocolate eggs, big and solid milk chocolate bunnies (where did that concept come from?), and oddly shaped forms of marsh mellowed sugar. EUREKA!

Working quickly, categorically harvesting only a few from each of theirs, I carefully filled my own basket placing the bulk of my score underneath its grass cover, preserving the overall appearance. Then carefully creeping out the screen door to freedom, and sauntering home, still carrying my own basket appearing similar to its holiday beginning; I was incredibly excited and happy! In that indelible moment of my existence I knew a success based upon serious planning and execution. Un-captured then, as I would remain throughout all but one of my many early life heists, I began that day a lengthy sojourn into the world of addiction: the challenge, the rush, the temporary satisfaction. Plus, crucial to the formula, the need to continue repeating these moments in variable forms to ward off that fearfully evil mindset we call boredom.

At birth, when formula was plugged into my mouth to satisfy my primal feeding needs, I was provided with my first and lifelong drug: SUGAR. (Whenever I use the word drug let it be known here and now, I am not reflecting upon the pharmaceutical industry. My definition of drug is that it is simply an addictive substance, or experience.)

Oh no! your mind protests, sugar is not a drug! Drugs are what either doctors prescribe, or nasty illegal substances! Sugar is sweet and everyone loves it!

Okay, so tell me if the following criteria meet your idea of what actually is an addictive substance or experience:

It is mood altering.

It is something which you crave when unavailable.

Without it there are withdrawal symptoms the least of which is physical craving.

And last but not least, you rely upon it for an effect.

Sound about right? Can you swallow this definition? If you have never felt a buzz from sugar then you are either unconscious or rare. In case the word buzz is unfamiliar to you, it is a word used by druggies which has entered the mainstream like many other "bad" words. Buzz is often found around the word sugar. And if you ask the students in our school system how they feel about removing the sugared drink machines, recent studies have proven you will hear talk that sounds very much like that of a junkie who will find their fix one way or another, legal or illegal. The fact that so-called health conscious americans have replaced sodas with bottled and therefore cooked until all nutrition is absent juices which are essentially sugar water, and candy bars with granola; also chocked full of sugar, just may be what's called in the world of addiction: denial.

Thus we have a Big fact which cannot be ignored: THE number one health concern for children in the usa: TOOTH DECAY.

Next in line: Diabetes.
'course right behind those: Obesity.

Hello!

Are we truly going to continue in ignorance? Are we really gonna continue to make our children sick? Do we really want to live this precious life addicted to something that is making us sick?

Since one of the simplest ways to identify an addiction is to attempt abstinence, try taking sugar away from yourself and your children. Personally, I'd rather take heroin from a junkie. At least the battle lines are clear.

Sugar wuz definitely my first drug. Just because it is legal, socially acceptable, inexpensive and easy to purchase does not automatically define it as non-addictive. Same categories are true for alcoholic beverages, and we do have a label for those who cannot give up that one; then guess what sugar turns into in your body. Check it out. The two substances have a lot in common. Since sugar is probably the closest readily available edible substance to mother's milk, it is no accident in the scheme of things that we all just want that oral satisfaction first; and in the end, often, last. Long before we reached for full body satisfactions, and again long after most pleasures stop, the desires of the mouth have ruled.

IN the 1960s, and even still, we all heard the preaching about the evils of marijuana - especially how it leads to the hard stuff. Try asking any junkie, clean or not, if long before finding the harder substances to abuse, they first consumed sugar excessively. If they are still able to eat and talk, they probably will let on that they did and still do eat lotsa sugar. Even 12 step programs often invite newcomers to switch their addiction to sugar while labeling their drug of choice cunning, baffling and powerful. I don't doubt the description, but can we just get it straight exactly what leads to what? Or if in fact anything is the leader. And besides, there are millions of professionally successful, totally together middle aged Americans who smoke pot and have never nor will ever be interested in the hard stuff. Just don't ask me for my research sources, these folks live within a government that can confiscate their land, home, vehicle, even child, and put them in jail for having a drug which has proven to be less damaging than the legal ones, and now even medically prescribed as beneficial. How many stoners get into public brawls, beat their wives, or puke all over the place? Worst common public offense, they fergit what it was they were sayin'. Ooops.

Back to my early start as a criminal addict. Nary been an early time in my life that I wasn't stealin' food, mostly sweets. I always ate massive amounts of sugar, except when starving myself for weight reduction. During starvation I discovered a documented fact, that dopamine is manufactured by the body as, I figure, it is Creator's gift to make starvation less painful. It works well. I still must stop myself to keep from grabbin' onto that dope - I mean!

From early childhood to age twelve I was consuming sugar at every meal plus any other time I could get it. My favorite sweet stuff was finally facilitating the natural consequence to over-consumption by creating the physical imbalance they explain away as a weight problem. Not every one gains weight when they over consume sugar, many people drop into a dangerously thin zone. For me, this excess fat coupled with the onset of puberty (ladyhood) drove my mother to haul me off to the doctor fer fixin'.

I weighed in at 128 pounds on my five foot almost two inch frame. In that baby boomer image conscious world, my pediatrician was obliged to drug me in order to correct me. Ahhhh, enter my first hard drug: methamphetamine, later known as speed, now as meth or crank ('cept the modern homemade recipe is not nearly as pure). Of all thangs, it was supplied to me by the very man who brought me into this world and advised my parents on my health for the first 12 years of my little life!

The societal message to this pubescent teen? Girls cannot become FAT women, else they are not ladies. Being a southern woman meant you must first and always be a lady. Boy did I forever blow that assignment! Yet I totally allowed my brain to be programmed with the meaning of it all. Fat girls don't have fun. Fat girls don't have dates. Fat girls don't marry. Fat girls are totally unacceptable, unattractive, and should not exist.

If not death, then what?

The fantastically unnatural feeling of control when one starves oneself cannot be ignored. Women of my generation were hungry to find the power that had been too long subjugated to the doll-like realm of hairdos, nails and push-em-up bras. To be able to bypass all primal instincts by denying ourselves food brought an unparalleled sense of accomplishment to us girls. Still does. And wow, how our peers and parents praise our efforts!

I was only allowed those diet pills for one month; by then my bod had been shrunk enough to be allowed freedom from dietary pressures. Plus, I did not care. I had found my next favorite drug: being in love. A full tilt parental nightmare had begun. They had trimmed me and redressed me and sent me out for the bidding. What they were not prepared for was the small town equivalent of James Dean to come riding up on his motorcycle and sweep away their now adorable little girl. It was eight solid months of completely passionately totally infatuated hormonally stimulated First True Love. yum. Between sucking face and another great lifelong addition to my oral repertoire, cigarettes, I cared little about engulfing sweets or any other food creations. I had love and touch and most important to girls of all ages, someone who found me attractive; and therefore, I had self worth. Who emerged into that passion ever cares that the worth gathered from the outside never lasts?

Together my first love and me discovered the peril of being programmed by years of believing I am FAT.

F: friggin
A: awful
T: thang

When he and I met I had shed the baby fat load and sported a healthy looking strong young body. And, had captured the adoration of the most wanted boy. We were mad for each other. We touched – no we did not do It. Woulda, but that's another story involving a late night in the woods, and Indians, and probably angels.

Anyway, one gorgeous fall day, he and I came around opposite ends of a patio corner and, spotted our love, and with hearts a-pounding, merged into each other. Fueled by great passion, he grabbed me up, hoisted me in his arms in that ever so loving way that I hope everyone gets to experience at least once in a lifetime. Love lifted me, higher and higher!

Butt!

Rut Row!

Soon as my feet touched the ground, here came my fist! Yep, I decked him! Laying there on the concrete, stunned and pissed, those blue eyes peering at me for an answer, he had become the first of many a lover to get sucker punched with no explanation! Just an equally shocked me, ready to flee, ashamed, and mute. Why? He had felt my mass, my heft, my burdening body at full capacity!

Alas, oh no, oh yes, as the way of the world always persists, and change remains a constant, my love life reality got crumbled and took my worth with it. That the wrecking ball operator came from within my family was unforgivable. My own mother had lowered the boom: either rid myself of my already too close to becoming a teen pregnancy horror tale with this wild young stud - tho success in our attempts to do the deed had been aborted......OR, suffer home imprisonment. Let's see: freedom with no sweet heart, or home with no phone, no television, no communications or visitations. I cried, I freaked, I cried some more. I avoided my honey and cried some more. After four weeks spent away at Girl Scout Camp, rarely escaping my mental torture, I finally told my dream sickle "it's over"; just like the Roy Orbison song I repeatedly played on my record player.

It gets worse, if losing your first true love due to your bitch of a mother aint enuff, in order to convince my ever so cute, seriously rebellious love sick pup to stay away, and that it must end; so that I could insure some freedom; which all in all he woulda translated into your mother is a bitch and we can sneak out to see each other; I knew I must tell him that I did not love him anymore. God help me, I did it! I lied not only to maintain mobility, but also to avoid claustrophobically provoked homicide; and to keep at least some feeling of control in my pubescent psyche which now recognized the fragility of freedom, of happiness, of self worth.

My friends hated watching my boyfriend's pitiful public tears. They turned on me for my betrayal of the one they jealously desired. Their distancing did not compare to what my mother had destroyed. Also gone was any hope of mother's ever being there for me as my nurturer, advisor or friend. Suffering alone with the big secret that she had provokated this emotional hell for me, I began developing a deeply serious attitude toward authority figures or any one else who dared to constrict me. In no time I'd stuffed my emotions so far that I ran many years into adulthood without shedding tears. 'Cept for the one time I bravely walked into the kitchen, watery eyed, because I had not been picked for something in high school and felt like the ugliest girl around. She took one look at me, asked me what was wrong, and then told me to go to my room and quit being stupid, and to diet more. Oh well.

The stuffing did not stop with just tears. Oh no. I stuffed my mouth and poor belly with countless pounds of chocolate chip cookie dough, usually homemade and sometimes when necessary for thieving that frozen stuff, bologna and cheese sandwiches on white bread oozing with mayo of course (ya aint southern if'n ya don't like mayonnaise), cakes, cake batter, twinkies, them new ruffled chips, you name it - if it was sweet or junk I ate it.

I stopped all crying and learned to shift my needs by using the only chemistries available to me: sugar, caffeine, nicotine, and my newly acquired best to date escape mechanism, alcohol. All told, not a bad collection for a 13 year old southern girl from the right side of the tracks. In fact I had gathered up pretty much all the tools available in the early 60's in Tennessee. If nothing else, I'm a fast learner, and a natural hunter gatherer.

By age 16 my weight had climbed to a whopping 145 pounds. In addition to food, I was now consuming as much beer as humanly possible while appearing functional to my evening cocktail always a little night time tipsy parents. On weekends nights, after a day of cheap wine or beer, me and my buds met at the Burger Chef or Shoney's, sent a guy to the bootlegger, and consumed pints of either straight bourbon, or when lucky, got slushies from the Dairy Queen and added good ole local down-home brew. On special occasions we mixed either moonshine or pure grain alcohol with grape juice. We called it Purple Jesus. A couple of glasses of that stuff and you at least thought you were in heaven.

A FAT daughter is a frightening spectacle for a mother whose world is based upon image. You see, my mother was an actress, and a local celebrity.

Probably due to her having to choose the battles worth wasting time over, I managed to be the only girl in kindergarten pictures in shorts always hiked up in the middle as chubby little legs will do, the only girl without a shirt in my neighborhood, until puberty, and the one who rushed home to put on jeans the moment school or church let out since back then dresses were mandatory. Being a tomboy wuz an acceptable category, probly cuz every one wuz ass-umed to be heterosexual.

As in my younger years, in high school I preferred the company of mostly the boys, with the exception of a few unusually wild girls. Labeled a slut because I drank and smoked cigarettes with my buddies, I managed to top off my public image with the shocking reality of growing rounder, definitely not taller. Hence, you have a mother frantically searching to correct this intolerable picture by finding what I consider to be the groundbreaking for all existing zillion dollar American diet businesses: The Fat Farm.

Duke University provided one of the first of these residential institutions; they called it the Rice Diet. Last I heard, they still do. Until some recent boo-boos and bad press, if you were a southerner with a physical problem yet unsolved by local doctors, you called The Duke. Those poor folks who went there for an obesity cure were living, or should I say starving, almost exclusively on rice and grapefruit, of course setting them up to need to return after a stint in the real world. All told, my mother found a total of three fat farms in the USA. Not bad for pre-google research. Eagerly sending in applications for my entry, yegads was she ever pissed when they all three refused me on the grounds that I did not weigh enough!

Forever tenacious, mother did not relent to the concept that I was not obese. At home sweets were being hidden. For a thief, that's a just a fun game. Meal quantity was controlled. Her obsession also became mine, as I bought into the concept that I was repulsively ugly and therefore worthless as a fat girl, well, except for my brain. When my mother invented the later to be called Atkins Diet, it of course worked for the time, as I lived on nothing but water and what we back then called club, whose club I don't know, salads: iceberg lettuce with eggs, meat and cheese.

Unbeknownst to mother and definitely uncontrollable for me was my alcohol usage. To render myself commode huggin' drunk as often as possible was my young goal; more important than being thin. Beer, cheap wine, champales, and bootleg whiskey do not fit on the low carb menu. These imposed diet regimens, plus my own fear-full of being ugly choice to just plain starve, paid off in keeping me from getting any larger, and I finished my high school years a drunken angry mid weight cynic harboring dreams of escaping to college and finding some kind of peace. Peace was the big word then, and oh yeah, I had also found pot.

Pot is a great herb in many ways. Back then it was inexpensive with few side effects, zero calories, pre dog sniffing days easy to hide, long lasting, and of course the communized beginning of a time in our country when it became the thread that bound the world of the expanding numbers of hip. Problem is, with pot comes the munchies. Sex, drugs and rock and roll kept me active, but pot kept driving me back to sugar. Though not very big, I never reached a thin frame those first quarters in college. The self image damage was already done. I considered myself totally unattractively FAT, unwanted and therefore unacceptable. My insecurities haunted me. I met a wonderful guy, but could not stay sober enough to hold him close. I still think of him as possibly the only one in a lifetime of intimate relationships who may not have been a serious addict. Maybe someday he will touch the pendant I gave him, decide to find me, and I will get to find out. May be.

Half way into my first college year, I was surprised to learn that students actually took those diet pills I had once known and loved. They dropped 'em to stay up and study. My first hard drug was in all the dorms and I was back in love with feeling the rush of speed in my frame! Didn't take long for me to become a full fledged speed freak. To sustain my usage, I dealt speed to the same fraternity boys who had previously found my overt wildness to be a bit much for their upscale image party ways.

One of the many times that my protective angels spared my crazy self from incarceration occurred when one of them frat boys decided to leave a message with my college dorm roommate. His message, written and left on the bulletin board was his latest order: twenty white crosses.

Too early in east tennessee for there to be much education or public awareness of any drugs; still very few pot head hippies; and most folks at least called themselves Christians. When I came back to the dorm and found the message that so and so wants twenty white crosses which was the slang for a low dose methamphetamine (you may know of the country song, "Weed, Whites, and Wine" - truckers liked them white crosses too)....I started preparations for my disappearance, figurin' I'm busted! Until my mate came in, beaming, so happy that I had not only found the church again, but that I was involved in a mission to supply crosses to those in need. Shew! I aint kiddin about angels.

When several whites did not provide enough personal kick, I graduated to the highest dosage in pill form, the black beauty. Not just my favorite color in those days, also my favorite horse story. Now my absolute love. Alas, when several of those beauties lacked my desired punch, powdered and relatively pure crystal meth to put in my nose and veins allowed me to live hyped to the max 'round the clock, sleeping only maybe one night per week. Thinking my self to be empowered, in control, massively intelligenting, little did I know that those blue light flashes I often saw were signals of brain cells exploding and that my precious IQ would actually diminish. By the end of my sojourn into what would have always continued to be my favorite high if my body coulda done it, I was quite sick.

After a very difficult withdrawal I landed myself at my parent's home for a summer recuperation. My digestive system was in total chaos, my nervous system was firing off madly and my psyche had sunken into bouts of paranoid schizophrenia. Butt, I was proud in the midst of it all because: I was NOT fat. That's what extended periods of speed can do for you - if you live. When I returned to school I had been probed, tested, placed on a bland diet and was occasionally able to eat without a lot of pain. My parents had lived through their daughter's first major detox without knowing it, while seriously wondering if I should be committed. If not for my brother's pleading that institutionalization was ineffective, I would still hold the scars, if I could remember to, of the methodologies made famous in movies like "One Flew Over the Cuckoo's Nest." They often destroyed the front of the brain on kids like me, or else inflicted so much electrical shock that memory of earlier days is sketchy if not erased. I am a protected miracle case for sure.

Thankfully clean from speed, I no longer suffered from paranoid delusions, but I felt zero vitality, had gained some pounds, and therefore my self image was at an all time low. I was a bi-polared mess with no diagnosis or clue that any of this insanity could have an inherited chemical cause. Ya didnt talk about that stuff back then.

Within days of re-entry into academia, I reconnected with a Vietnam veteran and home town friend. One night while tripping on LSD, we were lamenting about our aches and pains and he decided to let me in on his favorite form of relief: morphine injected intravenously. Those vets really knew how to make a girl feel good. One shot into the vein of preferably pure pharmaceutical morphine, or heroin or its prescribed equivalent like dilaudid, and I was happy to be in a human body with no worries or pains. Hell, I even loved everybody when loaded.

Now pushing on 20 years into my little life, still deeply depressed, still convinced of my ugliness, I was enamored with the needle and the relief it could bring. There were many journeys into psycho-delia, constants like pot and beer, but blues, our pet name for those little blue prescription pills of pure morphine, definitely ruled. Purely by Grace and not just a little help from my friends, I survived two unintentional overdoses.

As my tale continues, you will learn more of my mother and how only a few friends including the one I'll call morphine michael, knew of her power over me since I kept that like all other stuff – hidden. For now, be clear, the last thing on earth I desired for many years was for my mother, or her socially and politically powerful aunts, to be aware of my activities.

Without speed, staying in college had become a part-time effort. To catch up midterm, I had done some amphetamines to stay awake. When done with school, I popped in on michael to see what I could cop, plus I needed his injection assistance as my hands were way too shaky to hit up myself. Sweet guy that he was, and thinking me to be just overly nervous about school, not actually un-slept for three days and therefore in a very weakened state; he more than doubled the amount of morphine I gave him to shoot into me. Felt great! I immediately climbed up onto his bed platform built above the eating table. Them raised up beds were what we did in the one room hippie spaces.

If the record on the turntable had not stopped; and his girlfriend, star, had not been conscious enough to hear me, I would not now be.

What is that sound, michael?

Sounds like above us, maybe?

She climbed the ladder to find me turning blue and gurgling! They pulled me down, stood me up, iced me, slapped me, yelled at me, anything except call the authorities. Nothing was working and they were getting major scared.

Then as michael later told me, out of the blue his voice rumbled, "If you don't open your eyes I will call your mother!"

Shazam! I returned to the living! Apparently opening my eyes and giving him a stare like, how could you even say that?

After that one, I systematically controlled my usage to avoid a major habit or overdose. Continuing using morphine for many months 'til late spring, babying my buddies while they fought nausea from jonesing, spending hospital visits with my needle sharing colleagues sporting a joint and loaded works to share, I never contracted their hepatitis, and somehow evaded arrest on multiple occasions. I was surely blessed.

Still, when the phone rang in the days before caller i.d., and my mother's voice pierced - killing any buzz I might have achieved, there were always two questions practically perforating my ear:

How are your grades?
followed by,
What do you weigh?

Priorities.

At some point I could no longer keep it up. So many young people were either dead, sick or incarcerated. My real friends no longer came around since the disgusting sight of a zoned out junkie was too much for them. I was getting super paranoid again. My soul, I know, was speaking tho I cannot remember the words.

I left school and headed for the woods. Returning to my favorite childhood hideaway where I had pined over the decision to dump my first true love. Girl Scout Camp afforded me a respite; this time as a camp counselor; who thought she could recreate a sorely missed shelter. Eating meat and potatoes and lots of s'mores, swimming, singing, canoeing, and hiking was a brief reprieve into normalcy. At the session's end, I returned briefly to school, but my inability to concentrate or cope drove me away from each attempt that I made for several years to fulfill the parental dream of a graduated girl.

Next, I went for the adventure of living out west. Although a major culture shock, finding friends via drugs is always an instant connection. Keeping clear of the big two I had survived, I tested every new drug and held tight to a lot of the tried and true. All told, I suffered five years with constant diarrhea due to speed and morphined guts. This kept my weight at a tolerable level, and I slowly learned about healthy eating. Plus I held dear the digestive ease and aid which pot like no other substance provided.

During my 20's, 30's, and 40's I alternated between full scale partying and healthy living or a combination of both, if there is such a thing. And I never returned to the needle. For years my idea of cleansing my body was to spend a night dancing, sweating, and drinking either straight tequila or bloody marys, nottin like good clean white liquor combined with tomato juice and spices. What could be better for ya?

I must admit, for a time in my forties I did hang with a gang of guys who were awesome musicians and artists; and stained by addiction. They had a source for something I had never thought of again until then, blues, only this time in liquid drinkable form! Just could not resist. Like all drugs in my life, that agin ran its course, thankfully.

Back at age 28, I had suffered a debilitating' back injury which eventually led me to a doctor who tested my blood to review the functions of my organs. He explained that my back gave out because my adrenal glands were barely functional - not a surprise. While seriously low on funds and mobility, I ate very little and some how thinned into a slim weight which I held for most of my 30's and 40's. The only fat time I spent was when I got back into sugar and developed systemic excess yeast, a.k.a. candida. I lost the fat when I again quit the sugar, dairy, and wheat. And praise be, the phone calls from my mother asking what I weighed eventually stopped. Those pesky vaginal yeast infections also retreated, tho they wane in comparison to her.

At age 41 I was desperately seeking relief from an agonizing tail bone injury when I decided to attend a friend's birthday party. To ingest a fifth of tequila and dance all night seemed like an excellent method of anesthetization. When I landed on the dance floor on my left knee and had trouble standing, I should have gone home. Instead, after killing countless shots, stumbling around and straining my knee to incapacity, friends carried me out. When I woke from a black-out drunk ta my knee lookin' like it had ate a cantaloupe while hangin' out with a bunch of also wiped out and oozing ice packs! 'Twas scary enough puttin' together what probably had gone down. Then I tried to get outa bed and walk.

There's no describing the sinking sensation as I realized, not just that I was one legged crippled, but that I had driven to my last stand whilst in a totally drunken black out.

I COULD HAVE KILLED SOMEONE
... kept pounding my swollen brain.

That I could really have wrecked and killed someone made my already weak knees fold, my heart sank into a depth of dank only guilt can provide, and I threw up. Guess my gut hoped to expel the agony, but it was to remain. "The gig is up" resounded in my soul.

Not so graciously, but still, escaping one more time from the clutches of horrendous consequence and atonement, I have never since been drunk, nor have I driven while dangerously intoxicated. After that night I kept my self destruction to myself. A few years later I stopped smoking pot when my blood sugar moaned and my adrenal glands again weakened, this time from the mere stimulation of marijuana.

As in all years previous, chemical substances were entering and exiting my unstable existence when the hormonal insanity of pre menopause reared its evil head and wreaked even more havoc on my delicate nervous system. I was terribly anxiety ridden, so I did what every woman looking for that little helper does, I visited my hometown doctor. This time the opposite of speed was prescribed and I lived three years developing a hearty depend-dance upon the drug ativan.

Similar to the valium favorite of the women of my mother's era, I just figured, how dangerous could that little pill be, especially after all I'd done? Right, uh huh. Little did I know that those seemingly harmless pills came from a family known as benzodiazepine, considered by some to be just The most dangerous pharmaceutical from which to withdraw. Seizures and death are common when letting go of a hefty habit with those babies, also insomnia, severe anxiety, plus depression. Many years have passed since that detox, yet I still cannot look at flashing or florescent lights or ceiling fans without feeling dizzy and queezy.

Before ending my ativan run, my dear dear friend who had always battled with sugar, and in the end as a diabetic who never could quit the sweet stuff, died a slow and terrible death. Upon learning she had finally passed on somewhere far away where I could not be there to hold her hand, I sunk into a crying jag that would not stop. Sounds like a normal response to the loss of a close friend, but for me, who had experienced limited crying ever since way back in those terrible teens, I was in big trouble. After three totally out of control days I checked myself into a mental hospital and began treatment for depression - and subsequently ativan detoxification.

Although in some ways the scariest I had seen, this withdrawal signaled a finality which I welcomed. It was my only drug and seemingly would be my last to have to quit. Course I didn't know how difficult it would be to git offa those anti-depressants they put me on to keep me alive, so it was not the last, but sure thought it to be.

Upon my five day state imposed ready or not release from the nut house, still in the count down throes of withdrawal, I headed to my rural home. There I spent days in the woods in the coldest of a Tennessee winter, hiking so hard I would have gladly been naked of the sweaty clothing I carried. Shaking, crying, screaming, puking, and dizzy beyond belief, I fought the last of my way out of the womb of illusion and into the light of clear headed, clean bodied thinking. There alone in the woods I found again the core of my soul, my strength long ago stolen by so many substances, judgments and fears. I finally left behind my constant need for drugs to fix me. What most folks don't git is that the end of the usage is the beginning of the real work. It takes great courage, honesty, and determination to pull oneself out of that hole and into the present. Not only are the emotions immature, but the memories in the mind can be debilitating. Oh well.

As fer my first afore mentioned drug, recreational thievin', it peaked one day on Fisherman's Warf in San Francisco. I managed to work my way to the front where a magician was doing and selling tricks and magical paraphernalia. During one demonstration where he had laid out the pieces on the counter between us and was fast moving thru their usage, I deftly clipped a piece right under his nose without his seeing it. He looked at me with disdain, somehow knowing I was the culprit, but not seeing is not believing, and he had to keep moving. Not long after, feeling cursed by his anger, the decisive end came when a 99 cent pack of cream cheese stuffed into my back jeans pocket got me threatened with jail time. Okey dokey, had enough. Even in my tuffest of financial times, when I thought of just swiping what I seriously needed, I recognized that I'd played that one as far as it was gonna go. Any more and I tempt the punisher. No thanks.

Towing around multiple injuries and maladies due to my ruff and tumble lifestyle coupled with self-destructive abuses, my fifties also brought on a mentally and physically distressing time full of losses of career, love, family and friends. My hormonal, thyroid and blood sugar levels dropped way low. Plus my gyno put me on hormones. Afore I could say, "what tha?" I had gained a total of a hundred pounds!!!! From that slenderized size I had enjoyed for so long, my body weighed in (the last time I dared to look at the scale), somewhere above two hundred twenty pounds. SHITE!

Since that scale shock, my focus on healthy living and lots of healing has resulted in at least half of the weight being gone. At least, I say, cuz truth be told, I am so spooked by scales that I 'bout jump outa my skin if I somehow stumble into one. When my clothes git bigger, then I know my bod is shrinking and nevermore shall a number on a machine weigh so heavily upon me. Plus, someone out there always feels it their duty to apprises me of my size progress. Gee thanks.

As for sugar, rarely does it appeal to me, most times I've tried it there is an immediate nerve sensation in my nose and forehead, similar to that brain freeze from too much cold too fast, like ya git from ice cream. Only when it is gifted to me with loving and caring do I allow the sweet thangs. Then it usually feels good, in small quantity.

For now, let me say, I daily want for this excess fat to melt away. Whilst it is decreasing at a frustrating snail's pace, I will no longer starve myself. In fact, I eat every three hours to maintain blood sugar and adrenal stability. Continuing to study and adjust my nutritional intake while avoiding any diet fads, I continue to increase my exercise while babying and healing all the injuries, and I continue to know my body as it naturally is: strong and healthy.

As for my attitudes and opinions>
I am a sizest, bourne and bread. I hate FAT. I am incapable of looking into the mirror and totally appreciating my appearance. When I look at these new plus size models, while honoring their ability to feel beautiful, I sometimes view them with at least a twinge of distaste. And worse, I still sometimes catch myself wishing for

some quick fix, some fast way to slim up and feel good too.

Stupid thought habits……….no biggie.

After all those years of self abuse, I know I am not alone. You probably didn't lead the same life as mine, but if you are an american you are aware on some level, great or small, of the things I spoke. My heart goes out to all who ever even for a moment act in self disdain or destruction for any reason.

If you are not seriously affected by the weight of the world, someone you know and love is. Shoot, folks used to even give me a hard time when they thought my dog was fat, which he wasn't - just big chested.

Aint we got something better to do?

WILD NIGHT!
-a song by Kim O'Leary

Wild night, let me discover your end,
I have paved a weary trail to sit beside my only friend.
Oh wild night you shine illusory light
Saving me, grieving me, you snatched the butterfly.

Let me go you must abandon me,
I'm wounded by your fire.
I need redirection, sweet correction, love to take me higher.
I have sought for you and fought with you
Now I need no more warning,
My heart has turned my head around
My eyes await the dawning.

Wild night, you've got magnetic forces,
Spun me 'round, let me down, left me with no courses,
Wild night you wear the musk of a clear sky,
Danger I near by and you make the people cry.

Let me go you must abandon me
I'm wounded by your fire.
I need redirection, sweet correction, love to take me higher.
I have sought for you and fought with you
Now I need no more warning,
My heart has turned my head around
My eyes await the dawning.

Wild night, let me discover your end
I have paved a weary trail to sit beside my only friend.
Oh wild night you sing an empty song,
I heard it through, I danced with you, I wished that I was wrong.

Let me go you must abandon me
I'm wounded by your fire,
I need redirection, sweet correction,
Love to take me higher.
I have sought for you and fought with you
Now I need no more warning,
My heart has turned my head around
My eyes await the dawning.
I said, my heart has turned my head around
My eyes await the dawning.
I said, my heart has turned my head around
My eyes await the dawning.

My heart has turned my head around.

My eyes await the dawning.

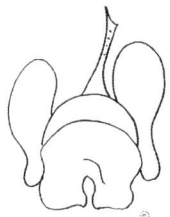

MOTHER DEAREST

My beginning attempts to find sanity back when seeking therapy meant you were absolutely nuts -course I was- but still, the stigma was thick. Countless therapeutic hours were devoted to one subject: my mother. Not just the biggest sizest I have ever known, she was truly a damaged psyche who passed on her thwarted emotional systems to the most sensitive of her children: that would be me.

Mother herself was born of a severely depressed Russell Stover's chocolate addict seriously poor excuse for a mother or grandmother or even human. Her greatest gift to us all was to allow my mother to pursue her lifelong dream. Unusual for the twenties, my grandmother was also addicted to psychic readings. When a woman in DC told my grandmother that one of her daughters was destined for the arts, and described mother, when the opportunity arose for her to begin dance lessons at age four, mother was the first student of two sisters whose New York City training and methods began preparing her for a life in theater, and fueled her childhood dream of becoming a New York City Rockette. In addition to their expertise, time spent in local theater provided early training which helped her to succeed all the way to Broadway.

Unfortunately, the primary love and stability of mother's formative years, her daddy, died suddenly on her 12th birthday. Her occasional, usually inebriated, accounts of that horrid day always included returning home from the hospital to the melting (frozen) punch bowl where her first "big girl" party was to have been. When that song came out in the 70's about someone leaving the cake out in the rain, I would think of her story. Although she spoke of his death on occasion, not until the late nineties, when she was dying of cancer, would I be let in on the "ah ha" that I sought after, the psychoanalytical answer to why she wuz the way she wuz.

Thanks to my brother's suggestion, while sitting around chain smoking, worn from chemo and radiation, she began writing down the memories of her life. The need to be known seems innate to most of us, and the need to feel a mother-daughter connection grew within us both during her last year. Still I was very surprised when she offered to read what she had written.

It began with her early theater experiences and the fascinating way her career started out at such a young age. She had me relaxed, enjoying her reading, enthralled with her story, when she delivered her expose' of the day of her twelfth birthday. First explaining how her religious, Southern Baptist father, Glenn, my namesake, had conceded to allowing a party of the finest of foods, plus permitted the rug to be rolled up for dancing. This part especially thrilled her, feeling his acceptance of her maturity and her chosen life profession in theater and dance. Truly a coming of age respect conveyed to his modern girl. They were quite loving with each other.

Alas, when she was getting ready for her celebration, the family was called to the hospital to spend the afternoon there, as her daddy passed away from a heart attack.

After helping clean up the cancelled party mess, my mourning young mom seriously needed nurturing. Practically crawling up the stairs to the bedroom area while outside the darkness laid away the end of a horrible day, she approached her mom's bedroom. Then, the icing on this cake of sorrow, the single most devastating event of her life occurred. As she entered the doorway she saw her mom, in bed, with the preacher…..sitting next to her, holding her hand as she wailed. At the sight of her 12 year old surviving daughter, my grandmother raised her hand to point at her, and screamed out,

"Why could it not have been her instead of Glenn?"

!!

Don't know what happened next long ago at that creaky old house. Don't know really what happened next between me and my mother as she stopped reading, lit another cigarette, and sat staring out the glass door. She never spoke again of what she had revealed, nor did she ever tell me how it all felt.

Stunned beyond time and space, I figure I probably got the dogs and went out for a walk. All I really know is that for me, the big Why? got answered.

The same woman whose original phone call informing she had been diagnosed with lung cancer no longer drew anything close to my blurted response,

"I'm gonna have to fucking take care of my fucking mother!"

Now don't cha go lookin too harshly upon me. That immediate declaration of my impeding caretaker situation was actually the only time I really expressed the terrifying complexity of being called upon to nurture one whose minimal skills in that area had been long forgotten in my own tortured mind. She really could be a major bitch to me whilst the rest of humanity saw the persona.

The one lifelong thread of stability in mother's life was that she truly was a talented actress. When she began dance lessons she also began landing small parts in the local Little Theater. During her grade school years she continued in her training and performing. Being included in the summer stock of the famous Barter Theater of Abingdon, Virginia was the coolest of her young achievements. Upon high school graduation she was allowed to head west to the prestigious school of the theater, The Pasadena Playhouse.

"At the Playhouse," as she often told us, "an aspiring actress must earn the right to continue study."

Which she did, to the completion of all offered courses. It was there that she went on dates with the later famous William Holden and trained with many who succeeded in theater, tv and film.

Graduating in 1943 with the stage name of Kay Turner, she headed for the only destination logical to a serious actress: New York City. Playing the game brilliantly, she got herself a job in the mail room of Newsweek Magazine, hand delivering mail to all who worked there. And she worked them. She had perfectly positioned herself to advance her career.

After landing some bit parts, yep even on Broadway, the escalating war actually provided her big break.

As we were all taught in school, there was a WWII Japanese woman named Tokyo Rose who broadcast propaganda to our soldiers in an attempt to demoralize and deter their efforts. NBC radio created a shortwave program to counter Tokyo Rose's efforts, and Kay a.k.a. Kathryn Turner, landed the part. She became the voice of America to many of our troops in Europe and on the sea. While on air, "Hi There Sailor" broadcasted the latest tunes interspersed with explanations of Tokyo Rose's misinformation, plus words of down home comfort. All this from the blonde beauty whose autographed "cashmere" pin-up picture went out to her fans. When chosen by Photo Magazine, pre-cursor to Look Magazine, as one of the top four "best of" the cashmere pin-ups, mother's photo was published along with Ava Gardner and two other lovelies. Newsweek Magazine followed with an article, including the pin-up pic, and a short bio. Curiously, school children studying WWII have never been informed of mother's radio show-one of those countless his-storical omissions about the role of women in US history.

As her career blossomed, her insecurities of a future without family bloomed. She foundered in her conflictions: continue as a single career woman or accept the repeated marriage proposals by her high school sweetheart. Shortly after the war ended, my parents married. Kay Turner gave up the theater to become an all american housewife. My father believed that women should be at home in the evening with dinner on the table, not out rehearsing or performing. In turn, my father's schedule as a pilot for Pan American Airlines involved worldwide travel which became unacceptable; and mother countered his career squelching demand upon her by insisting that he give up his other love and stop flying. And so it was that these two career-less and stuffed down deep bitterness of my parents left daddy's flight base city in progressive California for conservative Tennessee and the not atypical life of a small town middle class post WWII white family.

Except for a brief stint on the radio, mother's career in acting took sideboard until my brother was seven and I was three. During my therapeutic searching years, I always wondered just what happened when i was three. Every bad memory I had seemed to start around then. It was not until I was in my forties, and my brother simply asked, that we discovered the drama. In a nut shell, Daddy went flying. For six months actually. He just took off from his boring sales job and hit the skies again.

If you have ever studied the psychology of addiction, then the word caretaker will be familiar. Whilst mother was sitting around totally pissed and daydreaming of nights in New York City, going out on the town with men "who were like Greek Gods", not to mention, which she never did, but I know she imagined, the thousands of men drooling over her photos; little me figured i had caused all her agony and should totally forget my self and focus on how to make her happy. This role, coupled with equal amounts of rebellion against such a retarding reality, became My play - and i carried it the longest run of any.

When offered her very own television show - not as the stage presence of Kay Turner - but as the housewife supreme, she entered the screen world as the epitome of the 1950's dream. Similar to the nationally televised Dinah Shore (a middle of the state tennessean), The Kathryn Willis Show was all about women's interest: part cooking, part interviewing and the rest reporting on any story she could find. When the show began, television viewers had maybe two to three channel choices with no cable and no color. To have landed a television program airing 5 days a week, live, was a major big deal. Bigger, can you imagine the poise and control required to face the camera and perform daily? Add to that the constant local events and charities she either spearheaded or entranced with her presence, plus every public moment being recognized and approached. Kathryn Willis was, during her 27 year run, and still to some, THE local celebrity. She was a public persona who must always appear image perfect, representing the modern woman, happy to be hometown mom and wife and homemaker.

Let's now interject into this properly designed appearance of a perfect family, this here little miss never quite thin enough, often pretty darn bad and totally rebellious against all her mother stood for "li'l angels". (That's what my papa called me.) As they say in the south,
"If'n hit aint one thang hits anothern."
I always gave a gallant effort to maintain my role as her nemesis. Often there'd be times I'd be in the tv station near the end of her program when she was ad-libbing and she'd invite me on to the set. Every house wife and preschool or home sick that day

kid in the viewing area watched me over the years. That is, until my serious teenage years. Too many on screen battles and inappropriate attires ended my television career. Still mother prevailed with a long and successful run until, enter stage left, The Mother-F'er of all mothers, menopause. Any post menopause survivor will tell you that if nothing else, it'll make ya pray like a pig afore the roastin'.

With menopause mother suffered seriously severe high anxiety depression. Before that time she had managed to be what is called a functional alcoholic - usually not drinking too excessively even though daily, mostly nightly. It was during one of her change-of-life drunks when she informed me that the reason she imbibed excessively was to control her nerves. The tv show had to be cancelled when she developed an all over the body skin rash which even the docs at Duke could not figure out. Of course the good ole home town family dr. recognized "nerves" and prescribed, as the

Rolling Stones so aptly put it, "mother's little helpers", aka valium. She flat refused! Stating to him and who knows who else, that she would not become one of those drug addicts like her daughter.....so she drank. Don't cha just love the logic. Without work or public life, she drank to sleep, and to stay calm and to get through it all every day. After several of these horrendous, and albeit embarrassing years, my dad convinced her that either the drinking or he would go. It took a few trial runs, I guess you'd call 'em rehearsals, but she eventually took to sober life, with a little help from some sleep time friends. She finally decided to stick with the wagon after she overdosed on booze and sleeping pills and wound up in a treatment wing of the local hospital.

Calling in sick to work that day, I felt that one happen............miles away.

In treatment, for the first time since her childhood, mother unmasked, opened up, and spoke freely from the heart, and gut.

She spent two wonderful weeks getting to know and be known by her kind. She left there ready to publicize the beauties of companionship and verbal purging. One trip to an AA meeting where she was recognized and felt judged, and mother was back home well hidden, and herself again, just without the booze. Plus, that one AA meeting mother attended, there was one of the biggest known sobriety blunderers up front leading the meeting. Knowing too much about the woman, she had the perfect excuse, "That woman is not an example of sober! If she feels like a vacation, she just boozes it up until her husband sends her to the funny farm!"

Sober and maybe a bit wiser, mother landed her last part, a local human interest radio program. Even during chemo, the show went on ....'til just weeks before her passing. She had managed to hold onto her acting career her entire life. After all, every desperate but functional housewife is a fine actress. For mother, public life and emotional self control had been managed by capable denial-ability and by clinging to her one constant crutch since, yep, age 12, those little smoking guns. Guess we all come and go wanting to suckle for our comfort more than any other human action.

When first diagnosed as having lung cancer and told to quit smoking, out came her reply to the doctor, "The cows are already out of the barn, why close the door now? And besides, I might kill my husband.
"Until she was comatose, mother's desire was to smoke. Her hair or wig were always kept, her makeup always freshened. And believe you me, that was one funeral where I tried my level best to look presentable, to do her proud. As I greeted her friends and fans I stood strong- with a little help from "my friends"-as the proverbial daughter of Kathryn Willis.

Even though she stifled my spirit and creativity, stomped my mind and emotions and passed on to me the pain, anger, shame, fear and self loathing of a hard core addict; in those last months we were at times friends, confidants, and even mother-daughter, reversed when she would allow. With her passing I understood motherless child. We may not have been culpable, TLC not her strong suit, but she did always attempt to keep me safe.

That's a tuff
 heart breaking
 gut wrenching job
 when you got a brat like me.

Sometimes, I still miss her.

Often, I feel her protection.

We were each other's greatest challenge.

Perhaps I am a black widow
  seeking ever more vital
  sources of nourishment.

Perhaps I have drained you dry
and taken your life force
to sustain mine.

Perhaps.

But I think not.

Perhaps I am a gentle spider
spinning a hammock
to support you.

Perhaps I capture the early morning dew
on my lacy web
for you to admire.

Perhaps.

But you think not.

Perhaps we are both wrong
or right.

- Mary Ellen

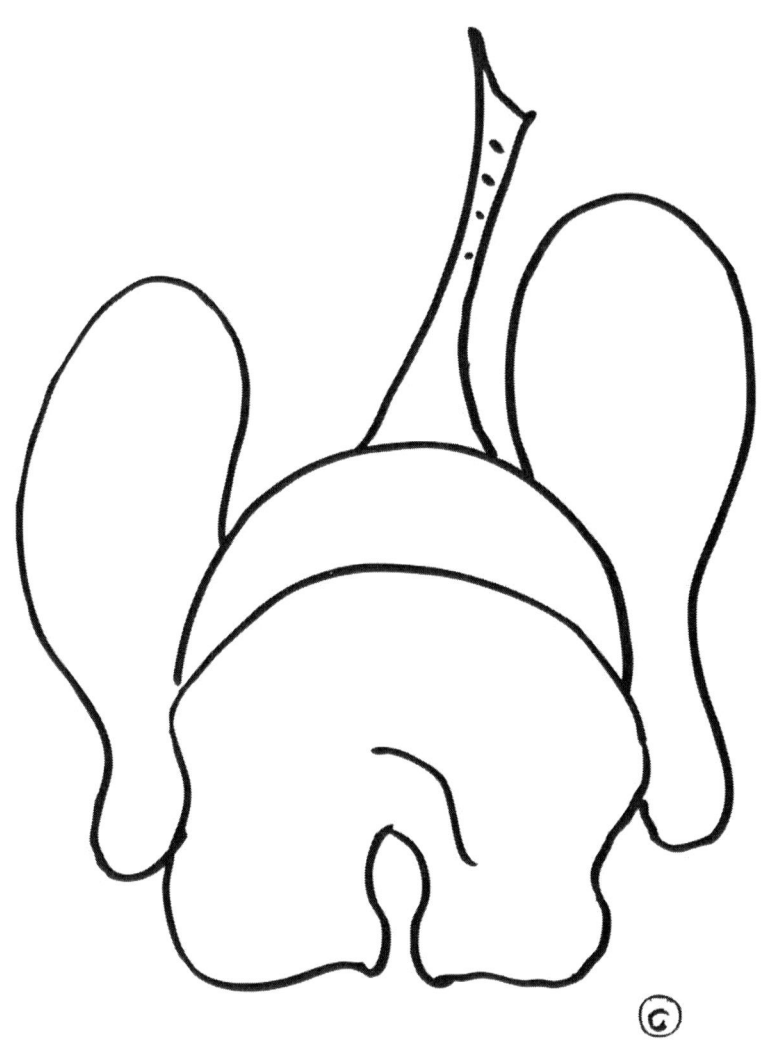

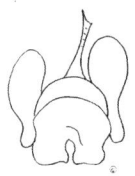

For Women NOT Only: BM-PM

Probably the greatest terror of my 60+ years on earth was the experience many women before me have called the The Change. Oh Cheee Waa Waaah! They weren't kidding. No other single bodily function changes a woman's life more severely than her hormones. I know there are those who say men go thru it too, but you won't find many women who believe it is equal. As for my poor ex, he begged me to ask the doctor for some calmers to my peri-menopausal self.

Before menopause (BM), and I mean before even peri-menopause, I was period time lucky compared to some of my friends, enjoying a short p.m.s. good excuse time to eat pizza and chocolate, followed by a short menses free of pain. When "they" say your clock ticks, "they" are right on it. At age 35 my hormonal world began to shift.

Not only did my periods get heavier and painful, but also, the torturer, PMS, reared its ugly face and began its nasty destructive deluge on my psyche as well as my little bod. I will never forget the day I was standing in my office when the walls started closing in and every pore on my skin burst with sweat. It was three days before my period and the beginning of a long claustrophobic journey into pure living hell.

That day was the first in seventeen years worth of PMS induced symptoms that subsided only at onset of menses. From age 37 to age 52 half of my life was spent certifiably insane. I could pinpoint the exact moment of ovulation. The egg dropped and took my mood with it. No matter what my activity at that moment: driving, walking, talking, whatever; when the chemistry changed, my basically ok outlook on life cascaded downward to "what is wrong with me?", then landed in a pool of "it aint worth livin."

When all this started it was mild and short. Within a few years I knew for certain that ovulation means con-foundation. And get this, when my periods moved into chaotic consternations of damn near bleeding me to death and I finally sought assistance from a- stupid me- older male gynecologist, he did at least ask, "What do you think the problem is?"

"Menopause," I replied.

"Menopause is when your periods stop!" His disgust bellowed upon me.

This obviously uninformed sad excuse for an authority did little research; and worse, gave little assistance, with zero info on the peri part. Since, I have personally come to know many women who started the change in this very manner.

In my mid forties I was barely mentally maintaining during what had become a nightmarish supply of pre-menstrual symptoms: extreme anxiety, depression, claustrophobia, poor depth perception, serious sugar cravings, the dropsies (when you cannot predict when your hand will just let go of what it is holding-very embarrassing at parties), confusion and more. Last but not least; I put in about ten well focused years of serious fornication without birth control, longing for the baby I could never have. Hormonal clocks do tic....

When relief of this psycho crap finally arrived with my period, I was flooded with pain, exhaustion, and a deep sadness, for once again I'd lost another chance to conceive, had again suffered another two to three weeks of horrid depression, and now had only two weeks to shake out of it before starting all over again. How nasty can you say the word: SHIT!? SHITE, SHOOT, SHUCKS, SUCKeeeeeeeeeeee.......

I think I tried every natural remedy known to women. After fifteen years of progressive desperation I once again approached the medical world for a solution. Doc then prescribed low dose birth control pills, plus ativan in an attempt to calm me. During the first month of hormone replacement I gained a total of 30 pounds. Yes, three zero, three clothing sizes, and thirty reasons to say this really bites! After the first HRT week I was freaking over the immediate weight gain, but the doc warned me not to stop the pills, instead to finish the cycle. Too afraid of being any more physically imbalanced, or more insane, the pills and weight progressed. Those thirty pounds were the same that coated me when I attended my women's group and heard that woman's declaration. Yep, the same thirty that started all this writing.

Next, I tried one of the more accurate methods of hormone replacement, and supposedly the safest. After paying $300 for a pee test to get a report on every hormone level, I bravely approached my hometown parents' doctor since I was again back in my roots world taking care of my Pa. This time, with the scheme that he write the prescription according to the hormone test; and that I would take it to a natural compound pharmacy to be filled. Poor man, he was the same doctor who figured out that my mother's rash was just nerves and tried to get her on nerve pills. Guess he and I just inherited the end of the story. Thus he went along with this progressive concept rather than fight another menopausal bitch from the same family.

A year went by of taking these "natural" meds. A grand total of 60 pounds later, still having periods and therefore PMS insanities, I chose to stop the pills and take my chances. With no added chemical in my system to keep me cycling, guess what, my body got to stop. Amazing what self healing takes place when you let it. No HRT - No period - no PMS. The damn shit was finally over!

My new gynecologist told me that after a year of not taking HRT, my hormones would stabilize and I would be able to get the weight off. I tried almost every diet known to somewhat sane americans. I gained more pounds. The last attempt at fad dieting was Atkins. Little did I know that people who are chemically pre-disposed to high anxiety depression often get very messed up by this eating system. Yep, the last diet I tried literally drove me crazy-er. Next, my thyroid went haywire taking several other organs with it and there I was, a FAT miserable extra hundred pounds middle aged woman who was really sick and really scared.

Have you heard the latest predictions? Seven out of every ten american women will be overweight when post menopausal? Worse, nine out of every ten over fifty men will reach the same category! It don't look good folks. And I aint talkin' sizist stuff. I'm talkin' health. These stats do give me great hope for the eradication of sizism. We surely cannot go around judging others when we're the same. Butt then, we are americans - we could, and we often do.

We'll get to the annihilation of that one later.

Before menopause I could not imagine a sane or stable existence. Now post menopause, I do pretty good. Who knows, with all the clean livin' and exercise I just might see my frame agin someday. Won't catch me holdin' my breath, or my happiness, at bay.

As for sanity. I am thankfull to be able to say it is now an easy choice. PM.
YEAH!

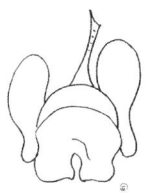

D-pressed?
 MAY BE O-pressed?

What a big business weight loss has become in this country! Just stand in line at the grab me section of every grocery and look at the magazines. Week after week, feature articles on dieting garnish the covers. Even certain cereal boxes declare that if you eat them 2 meals a day you will lose ten pounds. How very scientific. New network marketing companies pop up regularly with another seriously naturally this is the one campaign. Weight is not just big business, it is HUGE business.

Consider then, if all these publications, plus products and services ranging from books and pills to fitness centers and surgeons are so vested in the weight of the world, would they not also be quite miffed if we all decided to stop participating in their ventures? How many billions of dollars would we save and they lose? Imagine if you earned a humongous income from size-related sales, to what length would you go to protect it? Would you promote a fad knowing long range health risks are not yet determined and even likely? Would you work to assure the need for your particular product even if it meant fudging the facts? Maybe You would not, but are you sure others do not?

Just because you read it in print does not mean it is true. Publishing machinery does not have some magic button to stop the untruths. Whether printed on paper or cyberspace, neither is equipped with lie rejection capabilities.

When you see the photo of a bikini clad model that looks very much like someone you once watched dying of cancer while keeping their appearance as picture perfect as possible, do you ever ask yourself why you want to look like death warmed over?

In case you cannot answer yourself, let me assist. Maybe you are a victim of massive advertising campaigns which have enslaved the minds of the majority of americans. Maybe you want to believe that happiness comes from the outside instead of from the inside. Maybe you have so much time and money invested in the ideas being promoted that you do not want to give up or admit failure. Or maybe you have nothing better to do than purchase another weight loss product; paraphernalia designed to supposedly make sure that you become someone else's preconceived idea of beautification that someone else being the people who hook your attention with a plethora of techniques. Very simple biz technique: create the demand, supply the need, then make sure the consumer continues to believe. Believe the next and the next and The Next so called change in research.

Major depression, anxiety, and even suicide can result from self torture for the sake of weight loss. Health may be the reason for a person to drop extra pounds, but the methods used are embraced with little regard for the consequences. For instance, the current fad of surgically limiting food consumption has only recently begun to be studied at length and the initial results are not good. Previous statistics are being thrown out as studies such as the one by Dr. David Flum at the University of Washington find that the risk of death, yep extermination, not just illness, is much higher than we were originally told. Not a surprise to me. You cannot starve your body, or submit it to unnatural surgical methods, without running a risk. Read. Check the AMA Journal. Educate yourself before you kill yourself; 'cause after that, you got nothing left to lose.

While writing to offer the concept of sizism, I am reminded of the authors who have diligently attempted to open the minds and hearts of americans steeped in racism. Attending high school in a small southern town during integration was, to say the least, life changing. Now in the very same school where I spent my younger years, it is hip to be either black or a white kid who acts black. Amazing! But do we realize how limited our perspective was and still is? Black or white. We have slowly integrated into an acceptance which can literally be counted in the media – especially commercials and film. Asian Americans and Latin Americans are up on the count. Where are the Native Americans? And of course, due to economics, Mexicans are the new race to hate.

Still, you white southern girls, if you be white, don't be bringin' home a "colored" man for pa to agree to ya marryin'. Pa won't even yet call him by whatever color he might happen to be.
An if he be a she, uh oh.

Having lived as a southern woman who often worked in male dominated fields like construction, who was banned from playing baseball on an organized team after the sixth grade, and who watched many female friends get passed up for promotion while less qualified men got the job; I am well attuned to the sexism which still limits not just the salaries of women, but also their independence.

Fads of language, music, attire, and epicure repeatedly determine exactly where and when we americans let slide our dollars. Creating a circular motion known as the law of supply and demand, these cycles we choose determine the products which are manufactured for our purchase. Or is it the other way around? Do the "gods" of production and advertising create trends which become fads which get purchased? Whichever direction on the loop you prefer, the bottom line is that we are duped, doped and branded; then turned out to show, feathered in the latest fashion, spouting linguistic truisms, and swallowing the gourmet item of the year.

Need an example? Look at the ailing dairy market during the low-fat craze. until Atkins Diet became the rage. Low carb and nurturing cheese plus big ole juicy steaks cooked in butter mmmmm. Chance or design? You decide. Sure low fat, aka lite, still sells. Sells more sugar, sells more salt, sells more imbalance leading to more medicine and more weight and more diet programs.

Quite often our diet trends move too fast for research to accurately provide any real information. We saunter into, and even dance along, unquestionably programmed, unaware that our choices are seriously limited by what most folks call society. Few get the label right: BIG BUSINESS. We pride ourselves on being Americans, a democratic society in which each individual is an independent entity with choice and voice. If the doors to choose from are limited to numbers one, two or three, then where lies the independence? Maybe we oughta rename it american inter-depend-dance. Or at least call capitalism by its real name: corporatism. Sounds scary to some, but this is not a nasty view, simply realistic. I only hope to awaken us to our choices, educate us on our creations, and assist in basically calling it like it is; then we can best make use of it. It being the financial structure which determines our information gathering and spending habits.

Somewhere lost in this tsunami of societal sanctioning, somewhere washed up on a tree limb, sits the individual-at least for a moment; and usually only for a moment. If in fact some unusual someone functions from an incongruent stance, and if some anyone discovers them and appreciates their position, then that anyone will promote-even if just socially-that someone - in order to emulate them and once again a vision becomes a trend becomes a fad and defines the norm.

In 1996 when I relocated from Atlanta to the small town where this book was born, more than one someone suggested to me that my summer wardrobe was seriously suggestive and inappropriate. To me my attire evolved as a practical solution to the heat: cut off tank tops or t-shirts on top, men's shorts or pants with the waist band rolled or hanging down below my navel, and my feet either bare or in flip flops. Within a few years, there it was. You think maybe the style gods spotted me wandering the world?

Are we all awash in a mass of normalcy? Possibly we are, or at least the majority of us. Who in the daily world equation rules? How did it happen that body type determines almost every aspect of a person's life? Basic wants and needs like love, and money are directly affected by a person's size, possibly even more so than race, age, sex or even with whom you have sex. What a marketing gimmick run amuck!

'Twas not until my mother died and I landed the torturous task of sifting through her belongings that I found myself, one late night, sitting on the attic floor, sorting the photographic images of my life. There I was, at age six, posing as an angel for my first ballet recital; at seven in my brownie scout uniform, at age eight in my speedo holding my butterfly ribbon, at nine in my peddle pushers at Disney Land, and at thirteen in my cheering uniform. Suddenly I just fell backwards, surreptitiously banging my head as I realized that in fact I'd not been a grotesquely fat child. Rather, sometimes a bit chubby, assuredly muscular and quite attractive young woman. That night was absolutely one of the most revealing of my existence.

All of my formative years (let's just say before age 30), hating my self, not just my body, because I was taught I was fat which equals unattractive which always results in unwanted. My life was so very limited whilst hidden under this veil of self loathing created by someone else's idea of FAT. What can I say? My mother lived successfully amongst the stepford wives.

Did this sudden realization stir me into an epiphany of wondrous self love and appreciation? I wish. After the shock wore off, which took months, then came the anger, resentment and even hatred for the perpetrators of such oppressive beliefs.

Of course the figure head, my poor mother, did not act alone. The first authority outside of my home to attempt whipping me into size submission was my Brownie Scout troop leader who chastised me in front of the others for grabbing yet another brownie, the chocolate kind. I remember her snatching it from my little seven year old hands leaving only a dusting of powdered sugar on my fingers. She called me a pig and rallied the other brownies to laugh at my gluttony. Oh how i ran home to my mother seeking solace in the proverbial arms, only to be sat straight and shot clean with the concept that i must stop my unseemly behavior and realize how ugly i was becoming. How confused i was that these maternally produced goodies, material manifestations of love and nurturing, symbols of my inner craving for affection, were to be partaken of minimally. And most horrifying, how embarrassed i was that only I was hungry for more.

How did i survive when my mother chose from that day forth to limit my food intake and refuse my longing for the sweetness? I bucked up and created systems by which to procure the now forbidden sugar coated fruit. Number one plan: stay away from home as much as possible. Like I told ya in the beginning, the development of my aberrant behavior had a very strong foundation which held my maturation in abeyance for a long long time. If I have fought no other battle in my life, I have fought oppression. I knew from the git-go that in my world only one action equaled sin: the act of restriction.

The often quoted Marx stated that,
"Religion is the opiate of the people."
This less noted, at least for now, human being, proposes,

"Any thing that makes folks sick, as in junk and food in the same sentence, is the delusion, the anesthetization, and therefore The drug of the people."

It's ok, you can quote me. The american reaction to intensity is to find a form of opiation and seek separation. Unfortunately, we tend to remove ourselves from our very selves as well as our peers; rather than to leave behind the system which holds us down. While ignoring the innate ability to take responsibility for our thoughts and actions, we become unable to make our own choices. For information, we rely upon the news and advertising - actually the same thing-both bought and paid for. The majority display little curiosity as to the validity of these sources, or to the motivation, and the very real likelihood that our public educators - advertisers and the news medias - are those people who gain to profit upon our negligence.

There was a time, before our white male dominated industrialization of commerce, when the majority of women needed to be physically strong. Methods of keeping house, rearing children, growing and preparing food, were all aerobic and weight-bearing activities. There was no need to seek unnatural forms of exercise. But after WWII, the men in this country desperately needed to reclaim their territories. In factories, farms and even the home, women were relegated to the less physical duties as the men once again gained their place and reclaimed the control. Coincidentally, the social phenomena known as the housewife, became the norm. Where before women of wealth were the only wives with extensive time for leisurely activities, suddenly the middle class white american woman was being herded into a commonized corral of appliance ridden, appearance obsessed brand new version of the house frau. With brand new electrical devices, gasoline engine vehicles and indoor electricity and water, women gained some freedom from laborious tasks and cow-towed to this new house wife role. That, in turn, helped to alleviate the fear in our men that they had lost control. Tricky stuff. We were so happy to have our soldiers home and our world full of gadgets that we hardly noticed how many women lost the power they had assumed during the war.

As the advertised clue to marital bliss emerged as The look, not the make everything from scratch cook, Avon came a knockin'. Weekly trips to the beauty salon replaced washing and cleaning everything by hand. While coed evening cocktails replaced the naturally relaxing endorphins produced from hard work, male dominated businesses pushed coke, candy, faster faker "foods", to provide women a buzz.

Into this customized 50's hairdo and makeup world of the girly girl I popped, with a bod built for hard work and a total desire to realize the purported magical, not surgical, sex change my grandma promised if I could manage kissing my elbow. Spent hours trying. Even the sports world kept girls from most activities-except swimming. The spirits of water must have smiled the day I was born. I love the stuff. In water I'm weightless. Under the water, I am invisible, deaf to the chatter, and touched all over by its pacification. Ahhhhhhh.

When offered a chance to compete, if I would agree to swim on the water's surface, which was unusual for me. Us girls even got equal coaching when practicing, couldn't say that for many other sports. While I did bring home ribbons for the fly, 'twas the cool summer mornings spent diving into cold mountain water that molded a lifelong pleasure and release.

I also learned a huge lesson about our given image. Our team was gifted with an incredibly talented natural athlete, always number one in the girls' events, and the hometown hopeful to someday compete in the Olympics. Then came serious puberty, dating, and oh no, big muscles on a southern woman! She quit. Course by then I'd quit since usually not lasting at much of anything. But to watch her throw it away, woah. Made me ever more want to leave home and lift weights like the boys. Oh well, gave up on wasting my time on others' choices. Muscles still turn me on. Once in the early 90's I got to watch, front row, while Martini played a charity match. Pure poetry.

You can just imagine my reaction when the culmination of the 50's female suppression produced the modeling sensation of the 60's: Twiggy. OH MY GAWD! I was sick; I was disgusted. Every kind of advertising available proudly plastered that new - and still current - vision: the manifestation of starvation I'd longed to escape. We had progressed, if you want to call it that, from the voluptuous size ten of Marilyn Monroe to the muscle-less, titless, 90 pound weakling Miss Twiggy. The sick junkie look now appeared fashionable. The muscular healthy sized girls craved starvation, or rather the attention. What better way to keep women down than to entice them to starve, to look, and feel emaciated? Sickening, aint it?

Wish I could say we have escaped this self-destructive phenomenon. I can say that there has been significant progress. Magazines do now actually run articles of concern for anorexic celebrities. Muscle magazines now feature women on the cover. A few action movies have starred women; and a few of them actually even look the part. Although clothing models are still predominantly skinny, the fashion business has accommodated the actual market by offering "plus" sizes; a wonderful example of demand creating supply. The beginning of the "plus" time seemed so strange as I would open a catalogue advertising larger sizes for the "full" (as in ate too much?) figure, yet not one large woman was pictured modeling these now more creations. And true to the biz, designer tag switching has become the norm in even the cheap attire. They switch to the next smaller so that those who are enlarging can still say they wear a smaller size. One step forward, one step back. Stroke the ego and the women spend and strut.

Historically, in most cultures, excess body weight bore the sign of opulence. Now the opposite is true. Only the wealthy can afford the kinds of food required to keep our less active bodies slimmed. And only those with cash flow can pay to get exercised. It is as if we have flipped the coin on instinctual behavior. I cannot even guess where we go from here. We all know now that americans are gaining size constantly, with fat in the majority for years to come. Will we continue hating what is the norm?

What I can offer to those of you who wish to feel smaller, try oppression on for size. Feel it, know it, understand it. We may have come a long way baby, butt it aint over yet, not by a long shot. We've passed on to our children and grand children the same fear that has kept us locked away in our boxes in spite of our recent gains in size and for some in money. We are still boxed in.

Oh, American boxes! We hide in 'em, travel in 'em, stare at 'em, communicate by 'em, buy "food" already processed for us in them, and then….nuke it in one of 'em. Freedom?

O-pression

begets d-pression begets eat anything just to feel something besides boxed in.

Can you still think outside of them? For starters, try not swallowing everything you are fed,

especially in them.

ODE TO THE SKINNY
by kayo

some people actually hate you
 because you are not fat
some people actually resent
 you because you look like that
some people truly envy you
 since to them you appear at ease
those people don't see inside you
 where we are all just babies.

no one wants to hate a baby in the grocery line
everyone wants to poke at them
 and make 'em grin when they cry.
those pure little beings
 just reflect our sweetest thoughts,
but the reaction to someone looking thin
 when it's the way ya wanna be
it's enough to make us wanna throw up
or wonder
 if that is how
 you got this skinny
body
that we envy.

i sorry so much hatred is pointed in your way
i sorry you are questioned:
            "gone bulimic or got a.i.d.s.?"
i sorry 'cause it is all a front, a costume,
 a housing temporary
someday to be thrown away....

when we will all be equals
either rotting in our coffins
or part of the ocean spray.

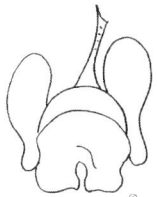

HOW DO YOU FEEL?

Whenever you read this, the statistics for those who are considered overweight will prove that we are a nation of people becoming enlarged, yet social acceptance will not have totally changed. You think the well advertised racism, sexism, classism, ageism and all the other isms are gone? The health problems which accompany excess weight are being emphasized now more than ever. We need help, not judgment, and certainly not legislation. An I aint talkin we, as in FAT. I talkin' we need help, all americans, 'cause we are prejudiced addicted numbed out, seriously in trouble half asleep beings who hold to our crap like we are gonna take it with us when we leave.

During the Viet Nam War my parents always replied to my ranting that if I want to complain, I should have something to offer in order to correct the situation. This really stuck for some reason, probably 'cause I hated everyone "establishment" and despised the idea that they could spout anything that sounded true. In good conscience, I cannot write a book about the pitfalls of hating others or ourselves because of our size or any other characteristic, without offering the best I know of correcting the situation. I have thus far accentuated problems like health and addiction. My primary concern is for the well being of all folks, not just those whose prejudices about, or whose size is harming them. We are saturated with the need to judge and compare ourselves and others, which can only bring about discord.

The modern media has proven that american consumers love to empathize, connect with, find solace and entertainment in the "real" lives of others. Even my once beloved weather channel is now basically a reality show. How's about some reality then?

Mother and child walk into dollar store. mother has in mind some household needs like toilet paper and laundry soap, hardly noticing all the other stuff. Child wants to touch everything, all shiny, grabbing along the way. Eat it, feel it, explore it. Difference in the two? Maturation and logic. Mom does not need or want everything in the store. Child does not yet have that discernment.

If child's maturation gets thwarted along the way while growing older, resulting in feeling denied and unnaturally craving what they should not logically purchase to eat, own, or play with, voila, you have a typical american consumer.

Finding myself, at the awesome age of 61, I am the cleanest, sanest, and happiest I have ever been. And slowly returning from years of being the fattest! Truly never before did I know these could coexist. When you escape the illusions of substance activated feeling and awareness, you allow yourself to just be who you are. Unfortunately, many of us believe that who we are is what we need to escape. Fact is, a person is not their problems, but rather a force far greater than the sum total of all their successes and all their failures. The core of our physical problems hides its insidious self in layers of conceptual illusions. What we think and feel we find made manifest on the outside. This is a factual quantum physics type reality very easily confirmed by observation: the simplest portrait of misery or happiness is sketched upon the molded face of the elderly.

Think of those you know leading an apologetic life, one filled with shame or the feeling of being a bother to other humans. Voila! Their attitude animates itself as a repulsive existence- one that repulses others. Then physically proves itself by conveying in actions, words, body language and good ole vibes that they think they are not good enough to exist. Saying to the world around,

"Do not support my existence. Do not take care of me, do not love me, do not fulfill my needs and desires, do not give your attention to me; even though these things are what I want and need -I cannot allow it. I am shutting the door."

This is what used to be called a self-fulfilling prophecy or self-defeat. In new age lingo, this is labeled manifestation.

Is there an escape from a nasty cycle? Absolutely. It is called acceptance. By accepting, taking in, what good comes our way; we communicate our desire to have, rather than to block, what we want. Now I am not talking about the love your stuff idea. Aint a gonna happen for me, especially when it comes to my body. Tried the let go one, the affirmations, even the pet yourself and love your fat one. You can imagine how well I did.

Existence is not a state of want or have, it is a state of being, it just is. To exist is to accept life, to allow self, to just be. When we judge and compare, as with sizism, we repel what we need and want, we repel each other - hell, we repel our own self. When we accept the fact that we are alive, when we accept having a human body with all the quirks and imperfections; when we allow ourselves the exploration into being just a unique creation during a very unique time; the inner turmoil really can subside.

Somewhere between popping out of the womb and adulthood, most folks lose a lot of their joy. One of those statistics circulating the internet said the average number of laughs an adult performs per day is 4-10, a child 110. Feel that.

Do we really want to live in fear, or angst, over the very personality of life itself? Do we want to miss out in each and every moment on the beauty of being alive because we are stuck in judging our latest action, appearance, or someone else's? Fearing what comes next? No wonder that we live unnatural and disconnected lifestyles. No wonder we grab for each eating concept spat out by the next vulture. No wonder we cannot remember the simple pleasures of feeling, choosing, enjoying, and laughing.

At the tender hormonally insane age of 45, my dentist informed me that my four upper front teeth must be ground to nubs and crowned. Seems they were beginning vertical cracks that could split to the root! Not only had my sweetened youth manifested cavities in most every tooth, but this malady, he said, was due to malnutrition. After many years of healthy living I was still paying the price of starvation dieting and drug usage. Still am actually. I often think I would be the perfect person to tour the country speaking to our youth about these dangers. Only reason I don't- they don't wanna hear it. I tend to go where invited.

We are living in the information age. Ideas concerning health, and especially diet, are so plentiful that most folks just pick the best advertised plan for their purchases. Misinformation and confusion reign. Why bother to figure it all out? Without good health, one's life is definitely impaired. Remember impairment, it is part of the definition of addiction. Without good health, quality of existence is poor; stress is high. Without a healthy body and mind, it is difficult to focus on any thing else. We all know this from experience. Yet most of us proceed in ignoring some aspect of how we injure ourselves. Not just a classic example of addiction but a very curious aspect of life in the USA.

While some of us believe that we eat, exercise, and generally do right by our bods, there is for me the pounding question: Why do we continue to cut off the very branch upon which we are sitting? Just putting in a good word for Mother Earth. Is it actual helplessness or have most americans lost the desire to take responsibility for our own actions?

Part of the natural separation of teens from their family is the attitude that everyone else is to blame for their problems. The assumption that aging corrects this problem has been replaced with the acceptance of our collective inabilities to emotionally mature. Working, voting, functional adults now place a phenomenal amount of decision making - and blame - upon our authority figure heads. Even when we elect them and pay their wages, we often know they answer to the folks who invest more in their career than we. When we cannot blame "them", then we actually turn on the very objects of our consumptions. If we drive it, put it in our mouth, sleep with it, inject it, or stare at it: is this "it" the perpetrator of our perpetual problems?

Who created "it"? Who manufactured "it"? Who purchased "it"? And who consumed "it"?

Yep, jus' li'l ole me and you.

As many publications have explained to us, our attitudes affect our health. Terminally ill patients who assume a decisive approach to their own care are faring much better than those who meekly do what the doctor tells them. Is this because they are better informed or discover methodologies not used by their practitioners? Not necessarily. It's in the mindset of responsibility: responding to what is happening rather than avoiding it; responding to our own need to be involved in our own health rather than allowing victimization by the problem or the treatment. In other words, we are at our best, and progress most effectively, when we are present in our own lives, welcoming our existence, and thinking clearly for ourselves.

Daily health practices are not just about our diet plan or workout routine, but rather about listening to the whole self and making educated choices. Without this, we are victims, people who are not accountable for themselves. We find reason in blame, solace in suffering, and rarely develop wellness.

So where do we seek assistance since we all seem unable to cut a clear trail in the forest of information that blizzards into our world every day? Let's start with our mother, nature that is. Health is after all a very natural state of being. It can, quite often, be achieved via natural methods.

First, the basics: when hungry-eat; when thirsty-drink ; when tired-rest; when energetic-move. The simple balance of creation speaks long for the basics. When thirsty we obviously need drink. Most of us got that one. Where we get lost is that the only substance created by mother nature for drinking is water. Flavored drinks are for pleasure. Water is for hydration. Watch a person who is dehydrated and you will see someone who not only feels poorly, but also cannot think clearly. Water is also for cleansing the systems. Our bodies have filtration systems and without clean water the filters cannot flush. Clogged filters contain gross nasty sickening stuff.

When hungry, some of us eat. What can I say, it's an american dream to be in control of bodily functions by ignoring their call. If you got it that you gotta eat, but wonder what to eat; ask yourself what would make you feel fed, your bodily machine fueled to keep it running and humming. Eat it. Then take note of how you feel. Yes, FEEL. Respondez' s'il vous plait. Do you feel nourished or do you feel yucky?

Illness and pain are the body's language of communicating its imbalances, aka diseases . Sickness is purposeful and necessary to the whole working system. If you eat something which makes you feel bad, time to decipher what is being told.

Since our mental venturing led us away from our primal and physical contacts with nature, most of us cannot correct our ill health by making choices based upon feelings. We need help. And since we know we need help, we turn to publications and other information systems which are created for mass consumption, and not individuals.

Health is not just about the body, and definitely not just about the size of a boday. We are a complete harmonious system comprised of physical, mental, and our spirit. The mental, which includes the emotional since even an instant thought precedes the actual chemical reaction sent into the system causing what we call emotion. This needs some serious concern. Why? Many foods can change the function of the mind such as the stimulating effect of sugar or the calming of your favorite "comfort" food. The mind in turn affects the body. If you are a person, like me, who tried the Atkin's Diet and wound up depressed and anxious, you are not alone as it is not designed for all chemistries. If you had your food intake limited by surgical methods and are stretching it back out to eat more, you are soooo not alone. If you are the acceptable norm in appearance, yet feel like crap all of the time, have some of those syndromes "they" cannot pin down like restless, fatigue, sensitive, and the whole bunch that all wreak of health imbalances. There are scores of good books about the physical and mental connections to how you are feeling and what your lifestyle determines.

When upset, I either eat more or don't eat at all. Nature's way when under duress is often to fast, since our digestive system, in fact most of our body's systems, are compromised when we are crazed. Putting food into a poorly functioning body is asking too much. So why do we sometimes eat excessively when disturbed? May be we seek that primal safety and comfort. May be, we make ourselves sick just to take our minds off what made us feel sick enough to eat in a way that makes us sick. To meet our needs in the most effective manner, we must get back to behaving with responsive clarity. If we address, respond to, this irresponsibility habit in our lives we will create great changes for the better.

For many years I suffered from a lousy self image. I'm not talking about just physical appearance, but my judgment of how I think and feel and act. This kept me in a self destructive pattern since I wanted to destroy that some-thing (which was unfortunately my identity) that seemed to be the source of my problems. A natural response to an unnatural state of being. I always chose intimate relationships with other screw ups as I feared exposure and judgment from anyone too together. Plus what better to place to ignore my own stuff than to focus on how messed up others are? I consistently functioned poorly. Fluctuating between bad action and inertia, I had only one belief about my capability to feel, think or perform well: not good.

Convinced at an early age that I could not be what I was supposed to be, then "i can't" became "i don't" and "i don't" further conformed into me that "i can't".

In a vicious and apparently unbreakable cycle fueled by harsh self judgments, I looked at myself, saw my fear, and hid. Alas, wherever I go, there I am, stirring around in my own crap. Desperate for escape from this shitty existence, suicide seemed the best answer. But it was not that I wished to die, just wanted to escape the person I believed I was.

I planned many suicides. Even "practiced" one. The day I swallowed a handful of downs to see whether I would need a bigger stash to do me in, was not the day I came closest to successful annihilation, just one of many. I am still here because my heart of hearts wants to be alive. I am still here because I let other human beings in on my need for help. I am still here because I finally responded to my true self. I stopped focusing on the messes, frustrations, and disappointments. We go where we put our attention. Finally, I chose complete responsibility for EVERYTHING happening in my life, in my head, in my body. Everything. Not a judgment call, not an open door to unleash more pain and blame, but a doorway to the freedom of choice. Simply put, an awareness that I do determine how my day goes.

In every bad pattern that keeps us down, there is choice. In every moment consumed with anger, we have chosen to fight with ourselves and our expectations. In every depressed moment we have chosen disappointment. In every wasted stymied by fear lay down and stop living or run hard from reality moment of my sweet little life, I chose to be controlled by reaction, rather than to respond with whatever action best takes care of me.

Don't freak yet, I am not saying we should be emotionless robots attempting consistently perfected action. Not at all.

What I am saying, or rather doing, is begging you to get into your own self and respond in each and every moment as you honestly believe is best for you (juss tryin' ta help ya here). Comparison to others is useless. Only you in your unique brain if you allow it to decipher, know what works for you. Having a hard time seeing clearly what to do? Caught in a bad cycle? Cannot see the way out? Pick a route, an action, which can affect change. Just one at a time. Attempt it, discern the results, continue. And appreciate the fact that you are still here and still making attempts.

After menopause and weight gain and massive heartbreaks and losses and years of bad thinking......I found myself stuck in a fat body and totally frustrated that none of the methods of eating I had before used to drop the pounds were working. The day I started breaking cycles of poor health was the day I finally saw thru the cycle of judging, blaming, battling, escaping, and decided to make one choice: to Feel Good. This meant that I would be literally walking through lots of physical pain from old injuries. It meant that I had to give up on giving up, escaping, blaming, complaining, fearing, frustrating, and generally self destructive behaviors. It also meant I would have to allow myself to decide moment to moment what felt best for me and to let go of my stagnated mindset of being a victim, even of hormones and other real influences, and be a smarter human being.

The cycle began to brake. From one little choice I found a feeling of appreciation and respect for myself. While no longer waiting for a thin body to make me look healthy and attractive and therefore proud, I found my own attraction in my own worth. If I can, any one can. Believe me, few functional humans can claim more intense nutsoidness than I.

The core of this choice, to be honest with and responsible to my self, has led to another and another. The cycle has turned into a spiral and is leading me out of my hole. Do I believe in white knuckle self imposed discipline to correct our unhealthy practices? Do I believe each of us wants and inherently strives to feel good? Do I believe that with education and assistance every one of us can make the choices that lead to better health? Certainly, I don't sit at a friend's dinner table and agonize over the servings - should or should I not, should or should they not???? Since I've found the real desire inside to feel good, just really don't want to put into my body what will make it feel like crap. Same response as when we learn we don't want to put our hand in the fire. Not super disciplined, just responding to my own needs. It is not that I go walking because I'm a super athlete, it is that feeling of awakening to the day by enjoying breathing and living and moving is so aaaaaaaaaaaahhhhhhhhh.

If you are, at this point, repelled cuz I seem to be one of those positive thinking let's all be constantly happy types you are barking up the wrong tree. I have bad days, really bad days and then occasional terrible days. If you are an american you are predisposed to bad days. We are a culture of the instant gratification syndrome. We turn on the pixels to find instant entertainment. We hop in cars to get to our destinations quickly. We have all these conveniences yet little understanding of things like the slow growth it took for a tree to get tall. It is a set-up to want instantaneous change. It can happen, but it often does not. Climbing out of a very deep hole, step by step, is an upward spiral, not a straight line to euphoric living. Every day that I look around and wish for more than I have is a day that I feel bad. Every day that I look back at what I miss is a bummer. If we can just know that our thoughts are our gifts to our selves, that we have choice of thought, and that change is a process not an instant drink, then maybe we can hold onto that spiral's line and not let go of progress in exchange for some erroneous concept of immediate relief. Every action does truly have a reaction. If you seek the quick way, you may just find failure faster. And get this, it takes less energy to simply embrace my days and all that comes along than to avoid them. Lots more fun too.

When my high school senior annual published, printed under my photo was the saying, "eat, drink and be merry." At the time I felt sure this referred to my excesses. For me now, it is a basic reminder to take care of my self, accept and ingest my existence and its nourishments, and appreciate what I have, here, now, for the moment.

When I desire the quick, I remember the quickening. Death will change everything quickly.

There was a song in the sixties which warned if you are not busy being born you are busy dying. In today's world, it's busy dieting. Just look at the word diet. It's die, as in cease to exist, with the symbol of a cross to finish it off. Respectfully, I realize that for some this cross symbolizes redemption. Practically speaking, the cross was a place to hang those who were accused of criminal behavior, a place to suffer and to die; a place where many years ago some very fearful and ignorant people tortured and murdered their own Living Master. If you wish to die-t by the cross of self deprivation, be my guest. Tho, I can pretty much guarantee you will not become a famous martyr, just another addition to the growing numbers of those who try unnatural methods, fail, and feel like crap.

In spite of all the advertised ways to defeat an overweight problem, americans are growing larger daily - to the point that it is the norm. The ever pervasive constrictions of dietary regimens are a national obsession. An ineffectual, brutally self abusive and, yes, terminal obsession. We are dieting ourselves into poor health and early graves. Yes we need better education and guidance on nutrition. But severe constrictions beget excessive resistance. We seriously limit food intake, then we binge, then we freak; then we repeat it all again. This pattern is not just harming our physical systems, our psyches suffer greatly.

Stress has become a household word and even a medical term. But what is it really? I think most of you would reply in definitions which only point to what we feel when we call it stress. Still what exactly is it? Lemme 'splain.

The degree of "stress" you feel directly correlates to the degree to which you do not want to be where you are, in any given moment.

For example, driving my car I wind up in a traffic jam. I get upset – "stressed"; don't like being stuck and don't wanna be there. How stressed I am equals how much I do not want to be there.

First, let's understand the basics of what is happening within me as I sit in this jam. The tension, the bodily reactions, are real physical responses to my mind's choice to dislike and wish to escape the situation. This is a primal reaction to fear or not wanting to be in a bad situation. My mind wants to be unstuck and arriving at my destination, or at least on the way. My body and emotions follow the mind's queue by responding with adrenaline which is a built in energy booster to give extra strength for motion, and makes my stuck body feel anxious 'cause it is getting the signal to be in motion but cannot. Plus the most important part of the equation, my mind has moved literally away from my body to a place somewhere else - like what will happen because of my stuckness, who will be mad or what will go wrong. This imagining of myself either thru wishing to be at my destination, or fearing what will be, not what actually is; when I am not there on time, causes a separation in a system which is perfectly created to be integrated. The whole me is no longer functioning properly, congruently. This is called discord, and becomes dis-ease. The more I imagine or desire to be away from where my body is, the greater the discordance. Warning signs like excessive fatigue, instability, and incapability are natural indicators that an improper state of health has occurred.

Acceptance of dissonance has entered into our accept-able reality so unquestionably that we make lists by which to measure the predictable degrees of "stress" according to events in our lives. In essence we are empowering and have vilified our desire to escape our own existences. We are in fact thinking in a way to release ourselves from being present which means being alive. This does scare the part of us that has some common sense. We seek correction because we have a natural propensity for staying alive.

We create correctional constriction as the acceptable human method for denying escape. With ourselves and anyone who bothers us, constriction seems to be the socially preferred option, such as institutionalization for those "others" and hiding out for ourselves. Yet the primal reaction to being limited is resistance by means of either expansion or its opposite, flat out shut down. While we fear our own reactions to constriction, we strengthen the walls of our cages,. Say what?

OK, in more precise and hopefully recognizable mechanical terms:
If you grok this, it will change your thinking and therefore your health - for the rest of your time here on earth. I swear!

First comes the natural reaction of fight or flight, so we desire to flee from an undesirable situation. Why flee? Because if we are socialized enough, we cannot fight (road rage is the fight part still unsocialized). This feeling to make flight in turn kicks in some form of self imposed restriction or constriction to keep us in one piece. This results in a very basic reaction called resistance. We naturally don't like to be caged, constricted, restricted. So we resist. The resistance against the constriction, is energetic compression, which results in further increase in reaction and a greater buildup of compressed energy. Once we build up energy inside we must release it or else the conclusion is explosion, breakdown, de-construction, or rearrangement of the internal system. This is the tricky part, while attempting to escape what is, if we do not balance both the pressure and our total self, we wind up harboring a potentially destructive force which these days is called stress, or we have little totally enraged cells trying to eat all the other cells because they need to eat their way out of their cage and this is called cancer. Discord within our own perfectly created system.

Time to chill on the technical and return to where I am stuck in traffic, needing to find a way to break the cycle. But, first, take a long deep breath, or go smoke a cigarette and actually enjoy your breathing since that's the main reason we smoke anyway. Those who began this new smoke outdoors only culture, did us all a favor. We get more sunshine, outdoor listen to the birds time, while the nonsmokers stay sitting inside. Plus, we meet other rebellious types and form bonds and have fun. And if you are wasting your time right now judging me, don't bother, it is just a way to not feel your own self, so might as well, like, flow with it. Actually, it is 108 degrees outside with a breeze that feels like it is blowing from some huge animal's mouth. I am sitting around in a wet t-shirt sipping on a mix of local honey, raw apple cider vinegar and ice-water. Sounds gross butt it helps with dehydration.

Breathe in, down deep, then breathe out, and agin....

I feel better.

Back to the being stuck. First correction to alleviate the stress? I recognize and own up to the fact that I have chosen to be in my car on this road in this very moment. Remembering who decided this. I am responsible for my presence here, even if, say, my boss sent me, I chose to obey. Second, since I chose this, I have choice to now accept my decision to be in my car at this very moment, where I likely cannot change the traffic. Next, I can bring my whole self fully present and find some enjoyment. When I lived in hot-lanta and got stuck, I either escaped along the side of the highway, turned around and went home; or I turned on country music for the simplicity and environmental noise protection, and alternately closed my eyes for a breath or two then glanced to see if cars were moving. Or enjoyed the surroundings. My world became again my choice, not a victimized nightmare. As I found myself agin, present, I was ready to feel life, instead of escape living. Valve opens, pressure escapes, breath renews, balance is restored, life continues, and stress is eliminated!

For over 40 years I walked in and out of the cage called diet, and away from most anyone who could not manage to be successful at one. Only recently did I finally decide to shut that door behind me forever. Every diet I have ever attempted brought with it a huge dose of hope. Hope that I would become beautiful, attractive, and happy. Hope that so many of my problems would just lay down and die 'cause I would at least look good hangin' on my favorite cross. Upon seeing the horror of a scale tipping past 220 lbs, I tried - for the last time- to place myself on a strict dietary regime for the purpose of weight reduction. Quickly recognizing the rebellion rising, of course to destroy the constriction, I became acutely aware of what dieters call this very response, failures or cheats. Somehow I knew this was my last diet attempt, and upon failing to maintain, became despondent. I couldn't help wondering if I'd continue to expand until my bod could no longer fit in my or anyone's world. Or just plain explode! Sensitive little me was afraid.

In a truly brave and honest response to total desperation, I admitted to myself that I'm an image freak. This further deciphered down to my gut level fear of being alone, unwanted, appearing unsuccessful and therefore incapable. To my friends, family, and business world: an eyesore, a pitiable failure, and so very uncool. And to the already very limited almost scarce world of eligible and desirable middle aged men, I ass-u-me-d myself to be an unmentionable, an uh-banishment, an avoidance.

Worse, oh yeah it can get worse, I'm excruciatingly aware of the necessity of touch. Not just sexual contact, but the very energy transference of touch, good ole TLC. So here came the catch 22 of my life: if I get the loving touch I need, I'm so affected, I drop weight. BUTT, without first dropping the weight, I can't allow the intimacy needed. SHITE. Oh so many long dark nights I reluctantly crawled out of the diet cage into the unknown. Where to, I did not really know. As a scientist I have been a lifelong experiment, but none has ever so disturbed me as walking away from the hopes of dieting. And if you have gathered anything thus far, you know I have my, shall we say, weak moments.

Weak moments have consequences. My years of self abuse consequented me with a very delicate physiological system which will not tolerate starvation or appetite suppression. I cannot even friggin' skip a meal without feeling like I've run outa gas. Lack of enough feeding results in adrenal stimulation which results in cortisol excretion which results in weight gain. OMG

One of the greatest beauties of this creation we are so privileged to inhabit is that, for now at least, the sun rises every single day.

In the light of day I knew I must release my obsession with size and restructure my focus to my own feelings and attitudes that make me unattractive. When I hate myself, I leave no choice for others but to do the same. All vibes are reciprocal. When I skulk around apologetically, no surprise that my attraction meter runs zilch. And when I fear, yes fear, the look of someone large, I fear my own plight and become, yep, we do become what we fear.

This weight thang coupled with all the other self loathing thangs, has been a long, way too long, struggle journey. If these words can shorten anyone's time struggling with their own self for any reason; or their judgment upon anyone, then, and I mean this, my crazed past life has been worth it.

For those who wonder about how to be balanced and healthy and free of stupidities, here is what do I do at feeding time. I make choices, educated healthy choices, determined by what is best for my body, not some one's idea of how to be healthy or thin. I study some literature; mostly I study my own reactions. Listening is also another lost american art. Not just to our bodies and ourselves, but try counting in one day how many times you get interrupted when attempting to tell a story, or just even get out a few sentences. Maybe that is why so many have turned to texting and emailing and social site posting, at least we can speak it before someone stops us and we cannot even remember what it was we were going to say.

I don't stress over food - especially when I am eating it. I don't deprive myself of anything I know is healthy for me. Some days I wind up just eating the same things because it is easy and no think and I know I am feeding the machine, not my addictions. So this is not a structure less nutritional scheme, it is based on what makes me feel good, which is usually what is healthy when I am honest with myself.

And best of all, the focus of my life is no longer on food and size. Instead my attention is on my life itself. It's on my own joy within and the love I can feel in my own heart every day when I allow it. Funny thing too, on days when I let myself enjoy myself and my own strengths and beauties, someone always tells me I am looking good. That's called empirical evidence.

As for the intimacy and naked fear of exposure, if I am not staring in the mirror, then I don't see my bared body. Solved that problem by covering my full length mirror with a cloth imprinted with a Janis Joplin drawing, so now I just see her having fun instead of all that stuff that seems to haunt me. Butt, if someone else chooses to view it, touch it, make love to me and my middle aged temple, well sir-reed, I say, "Let's get it on!" If I can choose to pick according to my aesthetic preferences, why then I guess I oughta allow someone else to do the same. Cheerleading tryouts are long over. Thinking my body is the reason another human would be attracted to me is passé. As my young friend Chris once stated, "Katy, you'd be a prize at any size!"

If you allow yourself the judgment free gift of choice, then please pass it on to me and everyone else. Let's let sizism fade into nothingness taking with it all those other pesky isms.

As I create my lifestyle from a clearer mind and heart, as I choose to be present in my life instead of attempting escape mode, I notice the effect ripples to everyone around me. That's how IT is, juss gotta let it be.

"Don't You Love Those Times?"
-a song by Steve McPeters

Now the world might tell you,
you're not worth too much,
but it's a world, that's so out of touch,
with what it means to be alive.

So wipe those tears from your eyes.
You've got everything, you'll ever need.

Now the world might judge you for the things
 that you don't possess.
It's all a game to try to make you feel
 like you're something less.

Heh don't believe in all those lies,
it's time to realize,
you've got everything, you'll ever need.

And don't you love those times?
When it's your heart and not your mind,
that shows you who you are,
cuz it don't have to be so hard.

Now your thoughts might tell you
 all the good things go to someone else.
You've known heartache and sorrow.
You're feeling sorry for yourself.

Maybe it's time you took a chance,
gone on that floor and started to dance,
you've got everything
you'll ever need.

Don't you love those times?
When it's your heart and not your mind,
that shows you who you are,
cuz it don't have to be so hard.

Don't you love those times?
When it's your heart and not your mind,
that shows you who you are,
cuz it don't have to be so hard.

Don't have to be so hard.

You don't have to feel alone.

Don't have to be so hard.

You've got a love that's all your own.

Don't have to be so hard.

Just remember who you are.

Don't have to be so hard.

You don't have to live so hard.

Don't have to be so hard.

You don't have to feel alone.

Don't have to be so hard.

You've got a love that's all your own.

Don't have to be so hard....

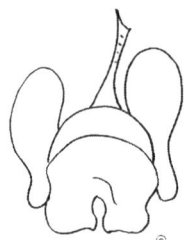

WHAT IT IS........

According to my original plan, this little book stopped at the end of the previous chapter, allowing me to return to living my life instead of re-viewing it; PLUS giving me the green light to publish and begin my campaign to end sizism. (be sure you get a t-shirt)

Wouldn't cha know, letting my bro edit my writing landed the biggest punch in this seven year itch to get published. He basically informed me that my A.S.S. wuz incomplete. So here we go bro – and you - if you wish to continue – an answer to the most important question of all: just what is my reality? Definitely not my size, my story, or my ideas. Definitely not what was or shall be.

In order to determine what is, tis always fun to make mitey sure what it is not....short butt sweet, here's a list of a few of my favorite illusions.

TRYING TO GET ENOUGH IN THE LAND OF PLENTY:

-workaholic: is there a more Americanized capitalistic lifestyle? Never mind that the rest of your life is in the toilet, you're making money. Absolutely the most judgment free way to live out an addiction in the usa.

-internet: we who use computers, and believe it or not there are still folks who do not, have all experienced the time warp when engulfed in the google. Do you know there are cyber wellness groups? These are not fer fixin' yer pooter. And if you feel you need one of these support groups, guess where ya gotta go to find 'em.

-sex: wish I could say for adults only. What better way to avoid real intimacy than by cloaking yourself in the intimate act?

-television: gotta be the single most popular mesmerizing anesthetizing time killing gadget to date. This illusion of social life is highly recommended for the lonely - so wonderfully non-confrontational. And now you can carry it with you wherever you go just like a companion that cant talk back.

-exercise: next to sex, it is the second finest method of producing our own dope-I mean. But when a runner won't stop running even tho her bones are fracturing from the impact, it sure makes me wonder.

-misery: not only does it love company, definitely often the only reason we have any, or anything to say.

-power and control: get this one down and you can have any other illusion in your world of choice!

-victim: ever try to help a friend leave a bad pattern or situation while simultaneously listening to their complaining and watching them return to what they complain about? The victim prefers not to find accountability in their responses, finding blame as their best friend.

-chaos: truly an adrenalin rush thang. The more messes you have actively demanding your attention, the less time to consider, and correct, just what a mess you are.

-lawn grass: say what? I've watched enough suburbanites to know that the stuff truly holds their obsession.

-concepts, beliefs, explanations: not just my favorite to sink into, but also to observe. Clinging tight to these does produce outright ignor-ance. Having a bad day? Musta been the planets. Need a reason to live? Any belief system will do. Cannot find satisfaction in your religious explanations? Musta been your parents or your past life. Just keep digging and processing and digging and anal-i-zing and digging for one more reason....'course when you find yourself in a hole, best thing to do is stop digging. Learnt that one on CSI.

Last and certainly not least,

-the big X: yep The BIG X – you've seen it replace a famous holiday's first name. You've seen it all over "bad" movies. Butt! Have you seen it as the biggest most destructive bane to human relations? X-pectations. Is it not the primary reason for disappointments which turn into pain and anger and hate toward others cuz they cannot satisfy our big X's? Aint it that the big X applies to me when I cannot live up to it and wind up feeling worthless which winds up feeling like I just wanna X myself?

Got the picture?

Time to discern instead of judge. Hatred stems from lack of understanding our true selves, the fear of another, and also the fear we are like the other.

Grok this: every addiction creates an illusion. All illusion is temporary. All illusive escape mechanisms are due to a lack of clarity and designed to escape living. In other words: it aint real! Even when a wonderful moment occurs in our lives, we attempt to repeat it, again and again. Why? Good ole fear of uncertainty. As we reach for and hang onto that which we know and believe we control, we literally grope for the dope of certitude. Yep, a lot like servitude. And guess what....that which you think is certain, 'tis not. Just another illusion.
****

To get a clear picture of what is, we gotta agin - this all forms and expels from my little life - go back to another of my early thieving stories. Yes. Growing up in a small southern town in the fifties meant very limited reading material and a library that had no computer or alarm system. Paper cards were used to indicate your checkouts. The process was free. So why another memory?

First, let me thank the open minded soul who donated a copy of Kahlil Gibran's "The Prophet" to our public library. I must have been about ten when I discovered its totally unusual message. Never having been checked out before, "The Prophet" felt so privately wondrous to me. Over a period of at least two years, I would get it, read it, return it, and then start all over again; after what seemed like an appropriate amount of time to allow some other some one time for discovery.

As you know already, puberty began with major angst for me. The need to have a book to which I felt a real connection became, welp, overwhelming. So, yes, one day when I was checking out several other books, before leaving the library, I smoothly sandwiched Gibran's between them, waltzing out the door with a charge that went much deeper than just adrenalin rush thievery. My soul was alit with an emergence to explore truth that no philosophy, no organized religion, no scripture, had ever accorded me. Since that time, and thru all my travels and repeated material downsizings, rarely have I been without a copy, tho reading it is often not necessary. "The Prophet" has always been my simple symbol of freedom where freedom counts – internally.

My mother once told me that I did not walk until I was a year and a half old; they were beginning to think something was bad wrong with me. Instead, she said, I sat like a chubby Buddha propped in the corner of the play pen, blissfully enjoying what they could not see. The next door neighbor's girl, born two months before me, and with whom I shared the pen, our homes, and my "best" friendship until she went after my first true love. Same guy – you know – the one mother forced away. Alas, that is so very past. Anyway, she, the neighbor kid, became mobile quite early, especially compared to me. As mother put it, "You sat happily while she crawled all over, even crapped on you."

Babies enter this world with open hearts and such a sweet countenance that we are reduced to smiley faced toe touchers whenever we get to be in their presence. Then as the world around us becomes too important, experiences shape us, we forget that connection to our purity. Apparently reluctant to forget my sweet non-worldly reality.... until curiosity got the best of me; then....Kapow! I took off exploring in a manner that required securing little bells upon me. Guess I tried to remain conscious of the not-here as long as I could. Actually, did pretty darn good at not being all here way into my fifties, when the need to accept living in a human body became a major issue to be solved, else life on the planet would become no more a possibility.

Upon becoming a babe who was ambulatory and seriously exploratory, it was obvious to adults I was also excessively sensitive, and still unlike many. Although not a nurturer, mother was a protector, and she sought to squelch my sensory perceptive capabilities. Very young I became very oppressed and, as you heard, sought relief in forms often addictive.

On the nite my horse died, when I was thirteen, I was home alone re-reading "The Prophet" in honor of Gibran's birthday, with no mo worry as to when it was due back in the library, if ya know what I mean. When the call came and a vast array of mental tortures engulfed me, reading Gibran's words gave me something in this world to hold to. Hope. Hope that one day I'd be able to understand and feel the wisdom, the joy, the knowing that guided his writings.

Today, and thankfully, every day, I am graced. It is truly amazing! I now know how to consciously go within myself and feel what scriptures describe. (like, "the kingdom of heaven lies within you" –The Bible)

With every breath we take, the life force of creation enters into us. From the first we take as a baby to the last we let out when we leave, every breath is full of the love, the power of creation, the gift of life itself, and can be for those who desire, a direct connection to the force of creation, a.k.a. The Divine. The very fact that my heart cried out to know The Real brought the Grace into my life which kept me alive during all those years where often I should have died or crossed into irreversible insanity. We all have our stories about being still here in spite of our stupidities.

My mother's view of my being odd had a lot to do with my personal makeup, not the core of my being. We are all the same down deep. The capabilities she squelched but could not destroy, such as to journey into what many call the metaphysical reality, with great effort and training and focus - eventually broke free and became my life's work. In that way we are all unique. Wherever we have talents or abilities, and with reference to our needs, as a human we all have a need to excel at what we do, and how that manifests can be as an awesome truck driver or dish-washer or mom or anything. For me, the many gifts I am blessed with getting to study and use are what tribal cultures label: healer, shaman, medicine woman, priestess, to name a few. To me, the names don't matter, except that people need them to find me if they choose. Having an ego about all the wild stuff I happen to do is counter productive. Folks hear the titles my work carries and immediately out pops that word, that idea, that enigmatic attraction:

POWER. They actually think I am powerful.

Do we feel so helpless and insecure that we crave and revere mystical power? Want to turn a rock into a rabbit? Why? Want to see blood pour out of a statue? Want to read minds? What for? Do you really desire to hear every one else's thoughts? Like you don't have enuff already pounding in your head! Do you really want to wave a wand and fix everything? According to what plan? Let's see, Your limited concept of how it all should be?

To know, to experience, every bit of creation, including us peeps, as naturally self healing; to foster allowing each of us to choose, and to assist in this clarification, that is how my work unfolds - naturally.

That idea of superhero helper, God send me an angel, send me my rescuer mentality, has resulted in a bunch of inept, ignorant, immature adults running amuk attempting to control everything. The result is painfully obvious. That big power we crave is called control. That real power is just energy, not something we control or guide unless we are miss guided, but rather some thing we allow to be. We are born to join it, not macho at it. Sure we have input, mostly we have need to allow the beauty of creation to show itself to us, to guide us, to be. Plus, we can wasa.

It is as tho we have lost trust in just plain living: feeling the élan vital! When all the idea-logical conflicts are released and we allow ourselves the simplicity of being – we can experience our natural state, which is, in fact, quite magical, as a sentient and responding, capable being. "flow with it" aint just a hippie slang. The river of life is not only flowing sweet, but also more powerful than any idea we can imagine. Don't forget, rivers cut thru rock.

Creation is magnificent in its diversity. No matter how dedicated each of us is to our life work, that does not define who we really are. We each have our very own DNA code. We are unique, each of us, in all of creation, the only one of our own style being.

"Every man and woman is a star," was how a man named Crowley greeted folks. I feel this. I know this.

I am happily enjoying what I do, worked a long time to get to be of use in assisting others to be alive and healthy, and shall continue in my commitment to being the best I can be at what I chose to do.

A lot of that training and practicing, what we call the hard work, was in the form of being my own guinea pig, my own test case. The injuries my mind and body have sustained and the fact that I can walk and talk and dance and enjoy is my proof that we do heal. I've toppled off horses, driven and been driven in numerous car crashes, landed wrong on diving boards, cracked bones playing football and canoeing, popped outa joint most of my joints whilst dancing, falling on floors and mountains and rocks, torn lotsa ligaments, been knocked out lotsa times, beatin' up or down depending upon how you perspective it, been stuck in a back brace for over a year and in a metal knee brace for six years. I have massaged with my arms and hands til I could not zip my jeans or chop vegetables. And with or without LSD, gone so far away that no one could reach me, for hours.

In all the ruff and tumble and cheatin' death did I feel free? For a moment. Like in that movie, "the air i breathe," where the main guy longs to know how the butterfly feels and what it recognizes when it comes out of the cocoon; we push and ponder and sometimes experience time's halting, placing ourselves in harm's way in order to accomplish a single moment of freedom and the awareness of right now as everything. At the time of death or severe injury, the world finally recedes to a less important reality. Then what? Then where are we? Is there an easier way? Or must we continue staring into death's face, or pushing our only body or mind past stability? Just like you, every day, I get up and head for the toilet, if you have one that is. Just like any body, I awaken with a need to feel free. In some ways we are all so very alike.

Definitely akin in our one universal truth, our heart of heart's reality. The thirst to know and feel the beautiful of who and what we truly are. Like Socrates said, "Know thyself." Not our capabilities, not our personalities nor our bull crap. The misconception that haunts us is that what we do is who we are and therefore our successes or failures determine how we feel about our selves and others. Just how wrong can one concept be? Ole Soc wernt talkin' crazy when he said "thy" self. As in, highest, most divine, absolutely real-est best of it all, undefine-able by ideas, flat out pure – and yes, free - self.

How do we go about knowing our realest, "thy," self?

Inside each of us lies a doorway to our Divinity. No matter how good or bad a person appears, they came into this world free of all ideas, all judgments, all fears -

these are all learned – we are all shaped by learning. Still, within every human being, there is a bridge to the infinite, the pure love, "the peace that passeth understanding." Not the peace we relate to as the absence of conflict, or the slowing down, sometimes one pointed, focusing of the mind. We all house the doorway to that which can and needs to be felt, to be known and not just believed in. It is not just a dream or temporary way of being. Too often it becomes the sought after never found idealistic "peace on earth" thang. Like where would that happen? And who would make it happen? And how long will we debate how to manipulate which power matrix to create it? And by which means do we make such an idea into reality? War. Force. No war. No force. Feed all. Fix all. Even be all.

The world to which we turn for satisfaction cannot provide it; it is an empty hole leading to more holes. The hunger we feel needs a source which is infinite and unwavering. We thirst for our true self, for satisfaction. We need hope and we need strength. Oddly, we humans must actually practice the enjoyment of our existence. Seems crazy, but it's true.

WHAT IT IS
is
my reality.

My primary focus. My need, my truth, my knowing; my ME. In that way you are just like me. If you hunger for fulfillment, if you need contentment, then know that this inner feeling, the knowing, of "I am o.k." is Reality. If you long to live in a world where the human internal wars no longer rule the external, which means that all of the isms become words the next generation'll be wondering what they were, like pill box hats. If you need to be ok with being alive, then know that it all starts right now, not tomorrow. My heart constantly longs to feel real contentment. My human self strives to see others feel free, happy and healthy.

And so dear friend, which you are if you got this far.... we read books to find answers which cannot be written.

Still, here we are. I am still here to tell you that your IT can be found and relished. By cherishing IT, then hopefully you may no longer want to judge, hate, or do whatever it is that still empowers all the isms. As we learn loving ourselves, we can also learn loving others. No one needs hatin' on. Every one needs lovin'.

This life is an invitation to celebration. And the best part of this party: It is come as you are! Might as well join in.

My sincere wish is that you and all you know may enjoy, not judge, yourself and others. May you give up on the endless and win-less mental battles. May you become fatigued of the worry over past and future, and find the lighter feel of this very moment called now. May you come to know that every breath you take is a gift - The Force is providing it freely, but not indefinitely. And not interchangeably - you cannot give your life to another. Which can then bring up the question, Is it really yours since you cannot give it away? Ahh, a conversation for another day.

Much more crucial even than what you accomplish or how long you live, is how it feels whilst you are here, no matter what is happening. How do YOU feel? How do I feel is about all I can handle, about all any of us need to handle in order to get goin' on a better world.

And it is all in the handling!

At least when I'm taking care of my self, I'm adding one clean clear brick to the foundation of a place,
a whole earth,
a reality,
which we can all be proud to have
allowed
to be
Created.

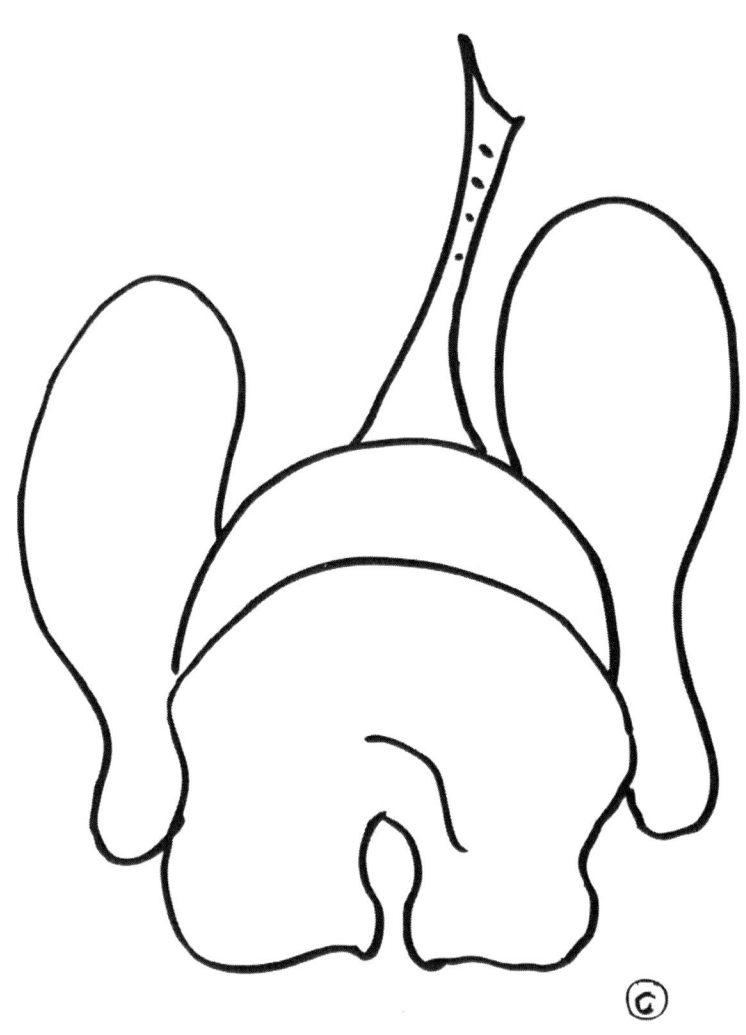

With all due respect to Yoda,
 cute as he is,
It's just not proper to say to some one,
That you hope that
The Force may be with them.

If The Force were not with you – you would not be here.

WHAT IT IS, is:

May You be with,

feeling,

recognizing

enjoying

appreciating

allowing

The Force

Constantly...........................

FREEDOM BIRD
by Prem Rawat

I have felt the urge
the freedom surge,
like you have.
Have you not the same fervor?
To leap beyond, feel the hover
to extend the wings
feel the winds
play heart strings.

Have you not imagined feeling free?
To feel
and see.

I have.

In my dreams flown above the streams.
Higher than I could climb I have reached,
felt, the sublime.
Like a bird beneath its wings
feel the winds on high.

I have, just like you
dreamt the dream
savored the brew.

I have lifted my head in endless pride.
Made freedom
my bride.

Upon the throne meant for people just like you and me,
I have commanded the soul
to be free.

I have, just like you, heard the heart
pound true.
My ears have rung with the message true.
My heart
uncontrolled
has leapt out,
my voice has quivered
spoken aloud.

I have heard again and again of the free space
felt my heart race.
I want the freedom bird within
to rise above
and fly within – the greatest of the uncharted space
infinite space
savored in slow pace.

Once again, I long
long to hear the very song.

Many a times I have heard before
that whisper within
for freedom bird to soar.

Spread your wings
push ahead in an unhurried pace
'til you have reached the endless space.

THANKS FOR THE READ..................
&

After seven long years I am happy to say: thank you............ to ALL of you who encouraged me, especially John and Elise, who provided me a hideaway to push thru to completion.

~~~~~~~~~~~~~~~~~~~~~~~~~~~~~~~~~~~~~~~

EH.........

LET'S ALL WEAR THE T-SHIRTS AND GO OUT AND FREE UP SOME A.S.S.

t-shirts are in natural and have the book's logo in red, on the front, over the heart.
T's can be gotten in all the available sizes, and can be ordered by contacting:

GREEN PEA PRESS at:
www.greenpeapress.com
(located in Huntsville, AL at the Lowe Mill Arts Center)

feel free to like them, and this book, on facebook

"don't try to make sense out of craziness. it is non-sense. mad is just plain ole madness"

- grandmother bear to little one

Now maybe ya can read cuntry, here's a little somethin so's ya can see if ya can speak it – hint: thars two of yuns.

A!

A

C?

C?

M R pigs

O no

O S A R

O.........L I B.......M R Pigs!

A Pigs!